Bedlam Among the Bedpans
Humor in Nursing

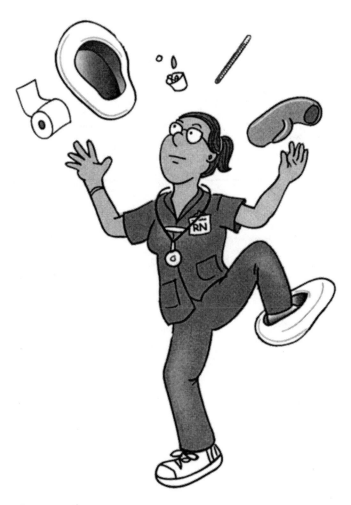

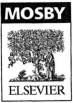

Compiled and Edited by
Amy Y. Young
Catalog Librarian
Wisser Library
New York Institute of Technology
Old Westbury, New York

MOSBY
ELSEVIER

11830 Westline Industrial Drive
St. Louis, Missouri 63146

Bedlam Among the Bedpans: Humor in Nursing

ISBN-13: 978-0-323-04524-7
ISBN-10: 0-323-04524-3

ISBN-13: 978-0-323-04524-7
ISBN-10: 0-323-04524-3

Senior Editor: Yvonne Alexopoulos
Senior Developmental Editor: Danielle M. Frazier
Project Manager: Tracey Schriefer
Design Direction: Kimberly Denando
Text Designer: Kimberly Denando

Working together to grow
libraries in developing countries

www.elsevier.com | www.bookaid.org | www.sabre.org

ELSEVIER   BOOK AID International   Sabre Foundation

Transferred to Digital Printing 2010

For Ken –

With Love and Gratitude

For

A Lifetime of Humor, Patience, and Inspiration

Acknowledgments

Organizing any book is a massive undertaking and this book is no different. Like all others, this book reflects the efforts and talents of many individuals. There are many people to thank for helping produce this book. Foremost are the writers of nursing humor, some of whom remain nameless, who have created this rich repository of literature. They have not only given generously their permission to reprint their material, but also have made suggestions and helped me locate other material that has added to the scope and dimension of this collection.

I am grateful to Yvonne Alexopoulos for her invitation to compile this book. Her wit, insight, and passion made the path to publication a pleasurable one. Danielle Frazier, Sarah Vales, and other staff at Elsevier also deserve recognition for their guidance and support throughout the entire process. Their professional excellence is only enhanced by their patience, skill, humor, and grace.

Finding many obscure articles would have been impossible without the help of many medical librarians. In addition, I gratefully acknowledge the assistance of Ms. Jennifer Thompson-Feuerherd, librarian extraordinaire, at the New York Institute of Technology and Ms. Antoinette Merges in the Interlibrary Loan Department.

Special gratitude goes to the editors of various nursing journals and their respective permissions departments whose help were invaluable in procuring those often elusive "permissions" to reprint.

Finally, I would like to thank my own family for being who they are, for tolerating my busy schedule and not taking away my computer. Their constant support and encouragement never cease to sustain me.

Introduction

At a reception last year, the President of the college casually asked me whether I had any plans for another book on nursing humor. At the time, I mumbled something incoherent, hoping that he would not pursue the subject any further. Coincidentally, that same week I received a call from the Senior Nursing Editor at Elsevier who asked whether I would be interested in working on another book on nursing humor because it had been 6 years since my previous volume was published.

A number of things have not changed during the intervening years. First and foremost, I am still not a nurse, and secondly, nursing humor is still poorly indexed, if at all, and the material that is indexed deals almost exclusively with utilizing humor as a therapeutic agent. After searching the usual bibliographies, indexes, and different databases, I again resorted to scanning 90 plus journal titles from 1997 through 2005 manually, with selective searches dating back to the latter half of the twentieth century. Only North American, British, and Australian journals were perused. Selections from 36 journals were eventually chosen for this collection and combined with material from 12 web sites and 6 books. All of the articles selected for this edition were published in the last 20 years, representing new material not published in my earlier books on nursing humor. Unfortunately, many outstanding pieces were excluded because copyright permission could not be obtained.

The following guidelines governed my selection process. All of the articles had to have been written by or about nurses. Each piece had to say something about the broad spectrum of the nursing profession, and it had to be funny or humorous. Since humor is still very much the lubricant in the solemn business of health care, I have made no attempt to exclude material that may be considered sexist or controversial. Rather, the goal was to have a representative sample of the rich array of writing styles.

The material is arranged into eight chapters according to common themes that all nurses will experience through the progression of their careers. The book begins with all the popular reasons why nurses enter the profession. It then describes how nurses view their patients, who are all "Lookin' Good But Feelin' Bad." In the third chapter, patients and members of the nurses' families discuss their adventures and misadventures with those in the nursing world. "Shall I Tell You What I Think of You?" dissects the special relationship nurses have with doctors. While negotiating through the maze of acronyms and the infinite variations of language, charting bloopers, and transcription errors, nurses are often tempted to ask 'Could We Start Again, Please?" The sixth chapter examines the rich diversity of nursing life, and the education of nurses is fully chronicled in "The Road You Didn't Take." The final chapter concludes by exposing the attitudes of management and how by revisiting the past the nursing profession reshapes its future.

Humor means different things to different people and it is not a substitute for clinically competent care. It is like a symphony to be played, a cipher to be analyzed, a bond to be shared, and a window to the mind. My wish is that something in this volume will appeal to nurses, their families, and colleagues. My hope is that humor will radiate through the windows of their minds or, perhaps, a large part of their minds as they sit back, relax, and chuckle at the bedlam of their chosen profession.

Amy Y. Young

Contents

Chapter 6
NIGHT AND DAY

It's a Fine Life 1

In our quest for truth since early childhood, we ask one of the most important questions of life with a 3-letter word, "why." As we grow older, we realize how important that word is and what profound implication that word has in each of our lives. It is only one of the myriad of questions that everyday life brings up, and many of them simply cannot be answered. We see our experiences through different mind-sets and try to come to grips with who we are and what is important in our lives. In truth, when we attempt to answer that all-important question "why," how we approach it is totally up to us.

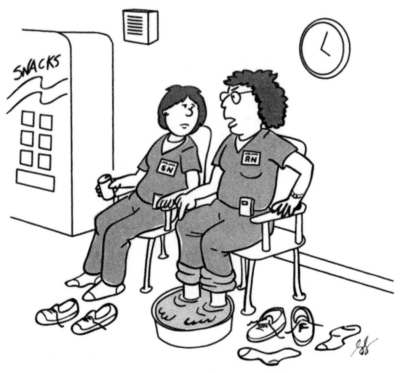

"Whoever wants to be a nurse ought to have her posture and feet analyzed!"

Top 10 Reasons to Become a Nurse

1. Pays better than fast food, though the hours aren't as good.
2. Fashionable shoes & sexy white uniforms.
3. Needles: It's better to give than to receive.
4. Reassure your patients that all bleeding stops...eventually.
5. Expose yourself to rare, exotic, & exciting new diseases.
6. Interesting aromas.
7. Courteous & infallible doctors who always leave clear orders in perfectly legible handwriting.
8. Do enough charting to navigate around the world.
9. Celebrate the holidays with all your friends...at work.
10. Take comfort that most of your patients survive no matter what you do to them.

Reprinted with permission. Retrieved December 6, 2004 from Medi-Smart, Inc. Web site: www.medi-smart.com

Top Ten Reasons to Become a School Nurse
Linda A. Vollmer

1. Lice is job security.
2. A bucket of ice is never enough.
3. Sing the praises of OSHA on a daily basis
4. Students who earn frequent flyer miles.
5. Paper pushing is good exercise.
6. Able to answer any sex education question without blushing.
7. Immunization records are always up to date.
8. Good Health is NO ACCIDENT!
9. Better pay, better benefits, better hours than any psychiatric facility.
10. Reassure students that bleeding stops....eventually.

Reprinted with permission. Retrieved July 25, 2005 from ©Love 2 Teach Web site: www.lovetoteach.com

You Know You're a Nurse When...

- You occasionally park in the space with the 'Physicians Only' sign, and knock it over.

- You believe some patients are alive only because it's illegal to kill them.

- You always follow the rules, but you're wise enough to forget them sometimes.

- You can't cure stupid.

- You have seen more moons that the Hubbell telescope.

- You own at least three pens with the names of prescription medications on them.

- You never get into an argument with an idiot, because they only bring you down to their level and then beat you with experience.

- You hope there's a special place in Hell for the inventor of the call light.

- You believe that saying, 'It can't get any worse' causes it to get worse just to show you it can.

- You wash your hands before you go to the bathroom.

- You've ever thought a blood pressure cuff would be an excellent gift for Christmas.

- You've ever spent more money on a stethoscope than on a car payment.

- You believe any job where you can drive to work in pajamas is a cool job.

- You consider a tongue depressor an eating utensil.

- You know it's a full moon without having to look at the sky.

- Eating microwave popcorn out of a clean bedpan is perfectly natural.

- You've been exposed to so many x-rays that you consider it a form of birth control.

- You've ever had a patient with a nose ring, a brow ring and twelve earrings say, "I'm afraid of shots."

- You've ever bet on someone's blood alcohol level.

Reprinted with permission. Retrieved September 16, 2005 from www.allnurses.com. Edited from the original.

You Might Be an Emergency Room (ER) Nurse If…
Michael Seaver, RN, NREMT-P, www.EMSCON.net

- You believe that 90% of people are a poor excuse for protoplasm…

- Discussing dismemberment over a gourmet meal seems perfectly normal to you…

- You believe a good tape job will fix anything…
- You have the bladder capacity of five people…
- You can identify the positive teeth to tattoo ratio…
- Your idea of a good time is a full arrest at shift change…
- You find humor in other people's stupidity…
- You believe in aerial spraying of Prozac…
- You disbelieve 90% of what you are told and 75% of what you see…
- You have your weekends off planned for a year in advance…
- You automatically assume the patient is a drug seeker when presented with the complaint of migraine, lower back pain, chronic myalgia (choose one of the above), a list of numerous allergies to meds (except Demerol), and the statement that the family doctor is from out of town…
- Your idea of comforting a child includes placing them in a papoose restraint…
- You encourage an obnoxious patient to sign out AMA so you don't have to deal with them any longer…
- You believe that "shallow gene pool" should be a recognized diagnosis…
- You have discovered a new condition that you call "hypo-xanax-emia"…
- You believe that the government should require a permit to reproduce…
- You debate which is worse, spaghetti and meatballs or pizza and beer, while performing gastric lavage…
- You plan your dinner break while lavaging an overdose patient
- You believe that unspeakable evils will befall you if the phrase "wow, it's really quiet" is uttered…
- You threaten to strangle anyone who even starts to say the "Q" word when the ER is even remotely calm…
- You refer to Friday as NH Dump Day and you don't mean New Hampshire…
- Your diet consists of food that has gone through more processing than most computers.…

- You believe chocolate is a food group...

- You take it as a compliment when someone calls you a dirty name...

- You say to yourself "great veins" when looking at complete strangers...

- You have ever referred to someone's death as a transfer to the eternal care unit...

- You don't think a referral to Dr. Kevorkian is inappropriate...

- You have ever referred to someone's death as a celestial transfer...

- You refer to someone in severe respiratory distress as a "smurf"...

- Your idea of a good time is dueling shock rooms...

- You have ever wanted to hold a seminar entitled "Suicide...Doing it Right!"...

- You feel that most suicide attempts should be given a free subscription to "Guns and Ammo" magazine...

- You believe that "too stupid to live" should be a diagnosis...

- You have ever had to leave a patient's room before you begin to laugh uncontrollably...

- You have ever wanted to reply "yes" when someone calls and asks "Is my (husband, wife, mother, brother, friend etc.) there?"...

- You have ever issued a "dead head" alert...

- Your favorite hallucinogenic is exhaustion...

- You think that caffeine should be available in IV form...

- Your most common assessment question is "what changed, — tonight, to make it an emergency after 6 (hours, days, weeks, months, years)?"...

- You have witnessed the charge nurse muttering down the hallway "who's in charge of this mess anyway?"...

- You refer to vegetables and are not talking about a food group...

- You have ever used the phrase "health care reform" to instill fear into your coworkers' hearts...

- You believe the waiting room should be equipped with a valium fountain...

- You play poker by betting ectopics on EKG strips...

- You believe a "supreme being consult" is your patient's only hope...
- You are totally astounded when someone from a NH is understandable...
- You have been exposed to so many X-rays that you consider radiation a form of birth control...
- You believe your patient is demonically possessed...
- You have ever had a patient look you straight in the eye and say "I have no idea how that got stuck in there!"...
- You believe that waiting room time should be proportional to length of time from symptom onset ("You've had the pain for three weeks...well have a seat in the waiting room and we'll get to you in three days")...
- You know the phone number to the local Detox Center by heart...
- You have ever had a patient say, "...—But, I'm not pregnant; I can't be pregnant; how can I be having a baby?"...
- You have ever had a patient control his seizures when offered some food...
- You carry your own set of keys to the "leathers"...
- Your idea of gambling is an ETOH level pool instead of a football pool...
- Your bladder expands to the same size as a Winnebago's water tank...
- Your feet are slightly flatter and tougher than Fred Flintstone's...
- Your immune system is so well developed that it has been known to attack squirrels in the backyard...
- You get an almost irresistible urge to stand and wolf your food even in the nicest restaurants...
- Your idea of fine dining is anywhere you can sit down to eat...
- You have a special shrine in your home to the inventor of Haldol...
- Your idea of an x-ray prep is a second dose of Haldol...
- Your idea of a CT prep includes Norcuron and a vent...
- You have recurring nightmares about being knocked to the floor and run over by a portable x-ray machine...

- Your nursing shoes have been seized and quarantined by either the Centers for Disease Control in Atlanta, OSHA, the EPA, or the Nuclear Regulatory Commission...

- You're able to tell the difference between a medical order and the ground around a poultry farm...

- You've been chipping away at your BSN for longer than most people take for a doctorate...

- Your idea of thawing the holiday turkey consists of an IV and warmed saline...(and if the holiday turkey you usually see has arms instead of wings and is sauced instead of basted)...

- You have ever referred to subcutaneous air as "Rice Krispies"...

- You have thought OD instead of BBQ when asked to get the Charcoal...

- You believe that a large part of your daily calorie requirement is provided by Tylenol, Advil, or Excedrin.

- AND FINALLY... YOU MIGHT BE AN ER NURSE IF...—YOU FIND HUMOR IN ANY OF THIS!!!

Reprinted with permission. Retrieved September 26, 2005 from www.nursinghumor.com. Edited from the original.

Celebrate! Celebrate! Dance to the Music of Nursing
Diane Sears, RN, MS, ONC

You Became A Nurse Because...

- It was "your calling," yet you aren't certain WHO called or HOW they got your number.

- Wearing a blue nursing cape was the closest you could get to flying like Super Man.

- You took the game "Operation" seriously.

- Whenever anyone in your family got bloodied, you fixed it because your mother became faint.

- You were fascinated looking at the plastic body over lays in your Biology book.

- The smartest women in high school selected nursing as their career choice.

- You looked great in white.

- Your dad told you that you could get a job anywhere, anytime.

- Your grandmother, mom, aunt or all three were nurses.

- Your boyfriend thought women in uniforms were sexy.

- You actually liked the smell of rubbing alcohol.

- You knew you enjoyed helping people and didn't bother to ask about salaries.

- You flipped open the college catalogue to Majors—and it fell open to Nursing.

- Everyone said nursing school was a certain strategy to meeting and marrying Doctor Kildare.

- You were good at darts.

- You couldn't imagine going to work in anything else but scrubs.

- You saw "Meet the Parents" or "Nurse Betty" and were sold.

After Being a Nurse for a While, You May Learn That...

- "T.O." stands for telepathic orders.

- Sometimes, the facts, although interesting, are irrelevant.

- Everything should be made as simple as possible, but no simpler.

- There is no substitute for a genuine lack of preparation.

- The careful application of terror is also a form of communication.

- Someone who thinks logically is a nice contrast to the real world.

- You have seen the truth and it makes no sense.

- If you can smile when things go wrong, you have someone in mind to blame.

- The trouble with life is, you are halfway through it before you realize it's a 'do it yourself' thing.

- You have done so much for so long with so little you can do anything with nothing.

- Stress can bring out the highlights in your hair.

Reprinted with permission from Oklahoma Nurse, ©2003; 48(2):31. Edited from the original.

So What Really Made You Become a Nurse?
Bina Goodman Simon, RNC, C, BSN

If my hospital got one new nurse for every time I've been asked "So what really made you become a nurse?" our nursing shortage would be over. And boy, would I get a "Bring a Nurse" bonus.

Of course, I have my own serious mushy answer to that question. Yes, I've wanted to do this since I was five. (What does a five-year-old know, anyway?) I've always wanted to help others. I've always enjoyed people more than numbers and computers…

Don't you think it's time we came up with something more original? Something that will finally stop people from asking this question ever again?

Something like, "I've always preferred getting up at 5:05 AM and running around like a chicken without a head for nine hours without a break for bodily functions, instead of getting up at 8:45 AM and sitting in a genuine leather swivel chair with a view of the skyline, drinking coffee and eating cake brought in by my personal secretary, for eight hours, including lunch and coffee breaks."

Or, if you are responding to one of your executive friends who's making three times as much as you are, what about a simple, "I needed a constant source of fertilizer for my Japanese garden."

Also in the tasteless category: "My family is in the detergent business and we always need, ya know, gross, foul-smelling, multicolored, deeply encrusted stains to test our products on."

Many nurses have joined the field (as in "battlefield") after witnessing nursing during a family member's hospitalization. Start your response with, "Well, when I was 15, Mom was in the hospital for three weeks." While you have your listener's rapt attention as he waits for a tear-jerking story, continue, "and I realized that nurses have easy access to sooo many narcs, know what I mean?" At this point, it might help to slur your speech a bit and make strange eye movements. You will never be bothered by that questioner again. Unless he's looking for a narc source.

If it's a personal story, as in, "When I was a child, I was hospitalized with a severe case of infectious meningitis," finish with, "so I decided that when I grew up it would be my turn to be the mean witch who jabs poor frightened defenseless sick kids with needles and tubes and strips them of their dignity—just like they did to me." Then give the widest, toothiest grin you can muster.

Of course, not everyone deserves such severe responses. Here are some benign ones:

"I never had any self-confidence and can't handle getting compliments or praise. What better field to enter than nursing?"

"I never liked wearing classy tailored suits and high heels, or looking chic and sophisticated. I've always worn drab, shapeless clothing and figured nursing was the easiest way for me to continue my personal style while still having a career."

Or, "Oh, I'd always felt nursing would be so rewarding! I mean, hearing the patients tell you <u>exactly</u> how they feel about you and the hospital every time you speak with them!"

"I'd always thought of the nine-to-five, five-day work week as humdrum and boring. I mean, who wants to get up, eat dinner and go to sleep the same time as your family and friends? And have the same days off? Nursing is much more interesting, with its unique hours and rotating shifts."

Along those lines, "They say 'Absence makes the heart grow fonder.' Well, with my schedule, I only see my husband on the third Tuesday of every other month. We've been married almost six years, and we're as much in love as the last time we saw each other!"

How about, "Oh, I just looove seeing the sunrise every single morning. Especially in the winter, when seven inches of freshly fallen snow looks like a beautiful carpet because they haven't plowed yet and there's no way I can get out of my parking spot. It's just indescribable!"

Or, "I really wouldn't know how to manage a lot of money. So I chose a field where I wouldn't have that problem."

Now, if all the nurses in the world would unite and give these and similar answers to that ever-so-redundant question, we could render it extinct. Then all we'd have to work on would be an answer to that irritating runner-up query, "So, why didn't you become a doctor?"

Reprinted with permission from Journal of Nursing Jocularity, ©1993; 3(3): 14-15.

You Know It's Gonna Be a Day When...

- The 11-7 shift tells the MI patient with organic brain syndrome, who repeats everything 30 times, "(Your Name) is going to be your nurse today."

- Your patient has orders for q 1 hour blood sugars and enemas 'till clear.

- Four of the nurses on your shift are pregnant, with due dates this week.

- The nursing assistant who just bathed your chronic ventilator patient in the next room cheerfully announces, "Oh, I see you got the endo tube out of Mrs. Jones…"

- Your patient has a doctor for every organ system.

- Your patient has an ex-wife, current wife and girlfriend who are all interchangeably short and blonde. And each one doesn't want the others to visit the patient.

- The new admission you got at shift change has twenty pills in generic form, none of which you ever heard of.

- Your patient, who has denied chest pain all day, responds to the doctor's "How are you?" with a pitiful look and says, "Oh, I'll be OK if this substernal tightness which radiates down my left arm will quit…"

Reprinted with permission from Oklahoma Nurse, ©2005; 50(1): 23.

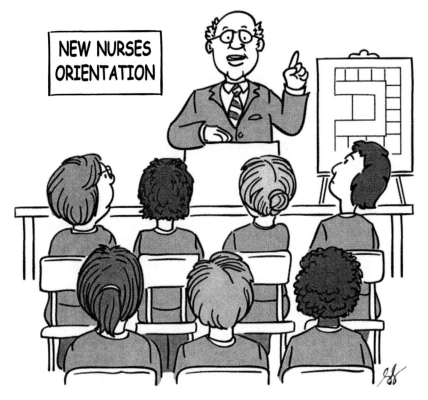

We have excellent benefits here…
at one time we even had a Valium fountain in the nurse's lounge!

Your Patient's a Nurse When...
Nancy Burden, RN, CPAN

- She makes her own bed—and her roommate's, if she can get to it.
- She reads her chart to make sure no one wrote "obese" in it.
- He records intake and output for himself and his roommate and takes his own pulse while you get his temperature.
- She asks if she's to be N.P.O. tonight.
- He takes out his own IV line.
- She knows her medications by their generic names.
- She apologizes for ringing her bell.

Reprinted with permission from Journal of Nursing Jocularity.

10 Signs You Have Become Obsessed with Home Care
Cynthia Blevins, BSN, RN

1. You automatically do home safety assessments when you're having dinner at a friend's house
2. If a relative calls seeking medical advice you first try to determine if they're homebound.
3. You can recite the location of every clean public restroom in the county.
4. When you sit down to write your annual holiday letter, you quantify exactly how many feet your son ran down the soccer field (without a considerable and taxing effort).
5. On your days off, you find yourself wanting to eat lunch in your car.
6. You can read a map better than your spouse.
7. Advertisements for vacation resorts described as an "OASIS" have lost their appeal.
8. You begin to feel guilty if you've been anywhere for more than 25 minutes.
9. You are extremely reluctant to throw away empty laundry detergent bottles and coffee cans.

10. You retrieve items from your purse using appropriate bag technique.

Reprinted with permission from Home Healthcare Nurse, ©2003; 21(5): 298.

You Might Be a Nurse If...
Michael Seaver, RN, NREMT-P

- You avoid unhealthy looking peoples in the mall for fear that they'll drop near you and you'll have to do CPR on your day off.
- It doesn't bother you to eat a candy bar with one hand while performing digital stimulation on your patient with the other hand.
- You've had a patient with a nose ring, a brow ring, and twelve earrings say, "I'm afraid of shots."
- You've ever bet on someone's blood alcohol level.
- You plan your next meal while performing gastric lavage.
- You believe every waiting room should have a Valium salt lick.
- You have your weekends off planned a year in advance.
- You have ever had a patient control his seizures when offered food.
- You know it's a full moon without having to look at the sky.

Reprinted with permission. Retrieved October 21, 2005 from Medi-Smart Inc. Web site: www.medi-smart.com

Top Ten Reasons Why I Went into Nursing
10. I love to wear white support hose.
 9. I get a kick out of arrogant doctors.
 8. It's more challenging than brain surgery.
 7. I get free latex gloves.
 6. The scrubs are so flattering to my figure.
 5. The world doesn't' need any more lawyers.

4. I actually like vending machine food.

3. Somebody has to train the residents.

2. I get to spend the holidays with my friends…at work.

1. I always wanted to say, "This won't hurt a bit."

Reprinted with permission. Retrieved June 27, 2005 from www.nursinghumor.com

You May Have Too Much Experience as an Emergency Nurse if…

Tom Trimble, RN, CEN

- The single diagnostic criterion in "had seizure in a restaurant" is "Had he paid the bill yet?"

- You don't eat while you drive to work because if you get in an accident you don't want to be a "*missed* café coronary."

- You don't eat before driving to work because you want to be an "easy intubation" if you are in an accident.

- You think Medic-Alert® tags make fine birthday presents or should be issued at birth.

- You see people in the crowd with stigmata of serious disease, and you quickly calculate if you could be recognized as an off-duty nurse.

- As above, but wish you had bought that CPR pocket mask you've been promising yourself.

- "Man down" translates to you as: Drunk if unwitnessed, Seizure if witnessed.

- Watching "film at eleven" on the TV News is like watching home video of all the ED and EMS folks you know.

- You realize that the House Officers and junior Faculty were born *after* you began your career.

Reprinted with permission. Retrieved June 6, 2005 from Emergency Nursing World Web site: www.ENW.org

Top Ten Signs That It's Going to Be a Bad Shift

10. The previous shift tells you, "Things have been quiet."

9. You walk onto the floor and someone from the previous shift says, "Is it that time already?"
8. You run into the pharmacist at the elevator, he hands you a case of Go-Lytely and says, "Here, this is for your floor."
7. Your phone rings 4 hours before your shift and they beg you to come in early.
6. After giving report, the nurse yells from the elevator, "Oh, by the way, they're 'pleasantly confused'."
5. While driving to work, every radio station is playing "Knockin' on Heaven's Door."
4. As soon as you walk in, someone hands you scrubs and says, "Here, you'd better put these on."
3. You come in and find one of the previous shift nurses openly weeping at the nurse's station.
2. The nurse about to give you report looks up from her notes and asks, "How many R's in diarrhea?"
1. There's no fresh coffee in the break room.

Reprinted with permission. Retrieved June 29, 2005 from www.poofcat.com

You Know You're a Nurse When...

You know you're a nurse when you won't touch a check with "voided" written on it.

Mildred Jones, RN
Summa Akron City Hospital
Akron, OH

You know you're a nurse when your child complains of a headache and you immediately think meningitis or a brain tumor.

Catherine Schneider, RN, CCRN
Children's Hospital Medical Center
Cincinnati, OH

You know you're a nurse when you find yourself signing your checks "Name, RN."

Susan Ladnier, RN
WellStar Health System
Marietta, GA

You know you're a nurse when you automatically assess the fontanels of every infant you hold at church.

You know you're a nurse when you ask the friend who just told you she has a cold what color her mucus is.

You know you're a nurse when you can eat an entire seven-course mean in 15 minutes or less.

You know you're a nurse when you can recount every blooper on "ER," but you can't remember the plot.

Helen McKay Wright, RN, BSN
Durham County Health Department
Durham, NC

You know you're a nurse when you use aseptic technique to open the ketchup bottle.

Star Allan, RN
Advanced Dermatology
Gastonia, NC

You know you're a nurse when your children ask if those cookies are for them or work.

You know you're a nurse when passing gas seems to be a good thing

Marsha Hatch, RNBC
Alamance Regional Medical Center
Burlington, NC

You know you're a nurse when you can discuss nursing practices while eating and not lose your appetite

Linda Patoni Diorio, RN
Retired
Lewisville, NC

You know you're a nurse when you look at the hands of the people you meet and think, "My, my, I could get a 16G (Jelco) into his/her veins."

Vicki Wise, RN, BSN
Mayland Community College
Spruce Pine, NC

You know you're a nurse when your bladder is full and your stomach is empty.

You know you're a nurse when a virtual stranger says he or she doesn't feel well and you ask, "What medicine are you on?"

Beatrice Law, RN, C
Ft. Worth, TX

You know you're a nurse when this actually makes sense: A person with Hx of CHF, DM, HTN, and NKDA entered ER with MI and TIA, had an EKG, CEs Q 8hr x 3, and a CT; then went to ICU, eventually to SNF, but went AMA.

Traci Thomas, RN
Bellaire Medical Center
Houston, TX

You know you're a nurse when your kids complain that you wrapped their Christmas presents with IV tape.

Amanda Darling, MSN, RNC, FNP-BC
Odessa College
Odessa, TX

You know you're a nurse when you can entertain your nursing guests using emesis basins for hot dogs, suction canisters to serve the beverages, and urine cups to drink from.

Karen Daugherty, RN, BSN
Self-employed research consultant
Pearland, TX

You know you're a nurse when answering the "how was your day" question over dinner leaves others wanting to be sick and you don't understand why.

You know you're a nurse when you can't watch "ER" without shouting back at the TV, "Wash your hands!"

Sally Leonard, RN
Methodist Willowbrook Hospital
Houston, TX

You know you're a nurse when someone extends his or her hand for a shake and you reach to take his or her pulse.

Virginia Lee, RN
Houston, TX

You know you're a nurse when you use five rights and three checks to give your child a vitamin.

Eileen Mann LaMothe, RN, MSN
Maurine Church Coburn School of Nursing
Monterey, CA

You know you're a nurse when you answer your phone at home saying, "Fourth floor, may I help you?"

Myrna Jane, RN
Memorial Medical Center
Long Beach, CA

You know you're a nurse when you set up a sharps container in your bathroom for razors and one in your kitchen for can lids and glass containers.

Laura Pagano, RN, MSc, CCRN
Naval Medical Center
San Diego, CA

You know you're a nurse when you trim your rose bushes with trauma sheers.

You know you're a nurse when you use a Viagra pen and don't feel embarrassed.

Karen Nosal-Fry, RN
Sharp Chula Vista Medical Center
Chula Vista, CA

Lookin' Good but Feelin' Bad

2

The nursing profession is a nurturing profession that requires strength, patience, stamina, and intelligence. Nurses invade the private spaces of patients whose lives are defined by diseases. The nursing profession touches them both physically and emotionally. Humor acts as the catalyst in enhancing the day-to-day communication between nurses and their patients by reducing negative tension and replacing it with a positive physical reaction. With humor, nurses can alter the various relationships as defined by their patients' illnesses.

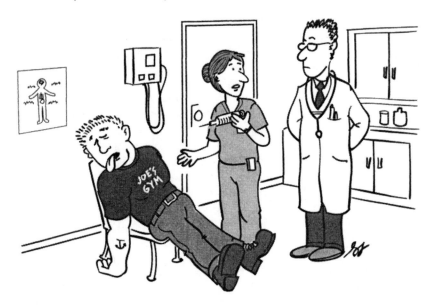

Must be the sight of my needle!

Blood Pressure
Jane Bates

So what is the deal about a bit of red stuff? At school it was a popular phobia. And if I did not scream or faint when Susan in the Upper Third

19

gashed her knee and bled all over the PE equipment I felt less of a girl, somehow. So I joined in and hyperventilated anyway. But however sorry I felt for Susan, and however horrified at her gaping wound, I was not the least bit worried by the blood.

Other people's phobias are always hard to understand. In one clinic where I worked, I had to take blood from about 30 people a day. And the old cliché was true. The bigger, the tougher, the more muscle-bound, tattooed and pierced a patient, the more likely they were to hit the deck at the first sign of blood. Especially if they were male.

'Nah, just geddonwivit,' they would say when you tried to persuade them to lie down first. And before you knew it they were draped all over you like a large ungainly scarf. I soon learned to dig my heels in and insist that they assume a horizontal position before I started.

Haemophobia—this aversion to blood—works in different ways. Some people, it seems, can cope with other people's blood but not their own. Like the stiff-upper-lipped soldier who looked as though he was about to have a baby, so contorted were his features when I was removing 10 ml from his arm for a routine test. I thought he would have been used to a bit of gore.

'Just a little scratch with a needle, Captain,' I explained, and he immediately turned a sickly shade of grey. 'But you are in the army…' He managed to mutter: 'It's the syringe,' before he drifted out of consciousness. Apparently it was all right with him if blood were spattered, oozing, or pumping from an artery. And it was all right if it came from another person. But his own blood? In a syringe? It was just too much.

I envy people who can pass out when they encounter their phobia. Except that I am scared of heights—and fainting would not be too useful at the edge of a ravine. But it does remove you from the situation long enough for someone to do something to help. And it generates sympathy from the general public, if not from the nursing staff, who will probably be cross with you for making the place untidy.

When my husband—a haemophobic—passed out cold in an antenatal class just as we were about to watch a film about childbirth, the midwives laughed.

Blood is not that bad. It is not the worst thing that a nurse will have to encounter. It does not really smell, it is a nice cheerful colour and is not slimy. If it was not for blood, all those phlebotomists would be out of a job.

It has also given us plenty of laughs over the years as we watched blokes who look like the Terminator cry out for their mothers at the words: 'Just a little scratch with a needle.'

Reprinted with permission from Nursing Standard, ©2004; 18(35): 22-23. Edited from the original.

Need You Ask?
Dale Blackston, RN

As I was filling out our hospital database for a new admission, I asked the patient, "Who can we contact in case of an emergency?" "A good doctor!" was the rapid response.

Denture Adventures
Jane Bates

In hospitals more than anywhere, teeth seemed to get themselves into trouble. In fact, if you were wise, you would no more take your best set near a hospital ward than you would take your pet lemming to Beachy Head. Years ago a colleague told me a toe-curling story about someone putting the wrong set of teeth into the mouth of a patient they were laying out. The patient's wife was impressed as he hadn't had a set of dentures for 20 years and she thought they made him look a lot younger. The person to whom the teeth belonged was not so impressed.

And who, as a keen young student, has not fallen into the trap of washing all the ward teeth in the same bowl and then being faced with the dilemma of which set belongs to who? It is like some bizarre 3-D jigsaw puzzle: 'It's alright, your teeth haven't shrunk, they just belong to the person in bed four... I think."

It is no wonder that patients, in my experience, have tended to be protective of their dentures. Keep them in the locker? No chance. They used to keep them in their handbags, in their pajama pockets, under their pillows, beneath the fruit, but never any place where a well-meaning nurse could make off with them.

I will never forget one patient of mine who, day and night, would keep her teeth firmly in her hand and never relinquish her grip on them, except at meal times. Then she would set them down beside her plate where they smiled at her serenely while she sucked up her mushy dinner from a spoon.

So we must ask ourselves the following. Are today's hospitals more denture-friendly? Are tooth outrages like these a thing of the past? I will leave you to chew those questions over.

Odious Odours

Jane Tyke

"You have some awful jobs, love," sympathised Mrs. Deaf, as I extracted a tonne of debris from her blocked ears.

She is right, although impacted cerumen is the least of my worries. We hear plenty about physical and verbal abuse, zero tolerance and all that, but what about nasal abuse? I mean the pungent odours that some people are determined to share with us.

Those of us over a certain age remember the TV adverts for Lifebuoy soap. Actors would hiss "B.O!" just out of the earshot of some poor soul, who was blissfully ignorant of their ripeness. The victim would then find a bar of soap in their locker and take the hint.

One hot day last summer I almost swooned at the collective odours emitting from a particular patient. It was a combination of greasy hair, fag breath and dirty clothes. Times are hard, but in this day and age it is tragic that some folk cannot wash under their armpits or change their socks occasionally.

The worst is when someone turns up first thing for a fasting blood test with the breath of Beelzebub. Maybe they haven't' heard that toothpaste does not have to be used exclusively after meals. Perhaps they want to punish you for their missed breakfast? "I am starving therefore you will suffer too while I keep talking in your face." My lung capacity has trebled as a result of holding my breath during such encounters. Consequently, I can now swim two lengths of the pool under water.

Strangely enough, I am not a complete wimp around bad smells. This country lass is regularly treated to a range of farmyard fragrances, especially from the bullocks in next door's barn. (Not the ideal ambience for a barbecue, admittedly, but rural life has plenty of other benefits to make up for it.) Animal aroma is more acceptable as the poor beasts cannot help it.

Being a garlic lover, my handbag is always well stocked with mints to mask the after effects. Second-hand garlic is not pleasant, as patients are swift to point out.

A chiropodist friend will not touch clients unless their feet have been thoroughly washed, then doused in antiseptic. She has a loyal following and commands an impressive salary from laying down the law like this.

Many women wash their hair just before going for their cut'n'blow to avoid disdainful looks from the stylist. Some even tidy up before the cleaner comes. Yet we nurses tend to avoid mentioning unmentionables like body odour, rather than upset anyone. It takes guts to tell someone that they don't smell the freshest. And if we suggested to patients that they had cheesy feet, bad breath or BO, they would be straight to the practice manager to claim victimisation. So we put up with it.

But I've come up with the perfect solution. I'm planning to install a sheep dip trough in the waiting room for patients to soak in while listening to soothing music. I'm going to sprinkle on the lavender oil and claim it's aromatherapy.

The patients will be so relaxed that a slightly neurotic nurse kitted out in full body armour and gas mask won't alarm them. I always knew there was a role for alternative medicine in the NHS....

Reprinted with permission from Practice Nurse, ©2004; 27(1): 54.

What a Weekend!
Margaret Clarke, RN

Called to the OR to help hold down a patient who was groggy from anesthesia, I put my arm over his chest and looked directly into his face. He was a good-looking young man I'd never seen before.

Suddenly he opened his eyes and gazed blearily into mine. Then he smiled and said, "I remember you. You're that girl from Vancouver. Boy, what a weekend that was."

He closed his eyes and slipped peacefully under the anesthetic. I'm still trying to live down the notoriety.

Reprinted with permission from Journal of Nursing Jocularity.

The Crisis of Today
Karyn Buxman, RN, MSN, CSP, CPAE

As a new registered nurse, I'd been assigned to work evenings in an intensive-care unit in a small rural hospital. Back then, as now, staffing was short, and I was the only RN working that shift. It was a quiet evening with only five patients, all of whom were sleeping or resting. I told the two LPNs to go grab some supper in the cafeteria and bring me back something to eat. Leaving me to cover the unit, they hightailed it out of there before I had time to rethink my lousy decision.

I pored over my paperwork, the rhythm of the beeping monitors playing their familiar tune in the background, when my nursing radar picked up an unusual noise that flagged my attention. *What the heck was that?*

I looked up from my charts into the room across the hallway to see a cardiac patient standing beside his bed. *Hmmmm, not a good idea.* Then suddenly, before I could even complete that thought, *whoom!*

His feet shot out from under him, his gown flew into the air, and he disappeared from sight!

Yikes! I leaped from my chair, shot across the hallway, bolted through the door and into the room. As I made my dramatic entry, I spied a giant puddle of greenish brown fluid spreading across the floor. *Nursing diagnosis: greenish brown liquid…body fluids…oh no! Poop!*

Too late, I was already hydroplaning across the spillage, arms and legs flailing to keep me upright. Always the optimist, my mind raced ahead with positive thoughts: *I'm going to glide across this mess, land on both feet and save the day!*

This, unfortunately, did not happen. Instead, my feet skidded across the fluid and then, *whoom!* I landed so hard on my backside, my head bounced off the linoleum. *Ouch!* I shook the stars off and rolled over to look for my patient. Spry thing that he was, he was trying to get up. *Boom!* He fell again. I tried to jump up to help him. *Wham!* I slipped again. He tried to pull himself up. *Whoom!* I scrambled for balance. *Wham!* With arms and legs splayed in every direction, we looked like Bambi and Thumper skidding on ice.

After what seemed an eternity, our eyes met, and I realized he was laughing. "It's probably not what you think," he said with a wink, and motioned to our putrid puddle. A Styrofoam cup lay tipped beside it.

Totally discombobulated, I couldn't understand what he was trying to tell me. "Huh?"

He shook his head as if to apologize. "I was hoping to hide my tobacco juice before you made rounds."

It took a minute to sink in. *Is this the good news or the bad news? Tobacco juice or poop: Which would I rather be wrestling around in?*

Not Just Window Dressing: Gowns as the Latest Fashion
Pam Johnson, BS, RT (R)

The door opens and onto the fashion runway steps—a patient. What that patient wears leaving the dressing room may surprise you. The classic medical joke from cartoons to get-well cards features the patient gown.

We offer two gowns to patients undergoing x-rays, other than chest and extremity, along with the instructions, "Please put these on in opposite directions," or "Put these on with one open in back and one in front." A patient's interpretation of those instructions often results in a fashion show.

The most prevalent runway activity involves two no-change changes—the patient who appears wearing a gown or two over clothes and the person who opens the changing room door with nothing on.

Others wear only one gown, open in back or front. We hear, "I thought you made a mistake," "I don't need two gowns," or "I thought you meant to give me pants."

Women appreciate a reminder to use the second gown.

Men present another challenge. If they can be convinced to use the dressing room at all, they usually resist the two-gown idea, preferring the open back. Some men don't fathom that other patients can't appreciate the view, even as the audience turns away in embarrassment.

Next down the runway come variations on the theme "tied at the back." The gown is tied at the neck like a bib, leaving the sleeves empty. Scanning down, the gown's neck can be seen, tied under the arms or at the waist. The gown may be open in front or at the side, sarong-like.

One man wore the second gown tied in the front with the hem pulled between his legs and the material tucked in at the waist, creating shorts.

I've witnessed heads poking through armholes in an asymmetric fashion that would make designer Issai Miyake proud.

One woman donned a gown, front open, and sat in the waiting room using the other gown as a blanket—over her legs.

Some patients put both gowns on the same way so that they gape revealingly open. These patients often claim that they thought we gave them just another dumb hospital instruction.

We always are alert for the patients, usually men, who disrobe with the door open, if they are not allowed to undress in the hall. When women do this, they laugh in embarrassment at the way the hospital makes them lose all modesty.

Men give me mock looks of disappointment, like I'm ruining their fun.

People frequently enter the exam room and start to shed their gowns. They look amazed when we ask them not to disrobe and often comment, "X-rays can go through this?"

I can't believe that they seem to believe their bodies are less dense than thin cloth.

Our department once used three-armhole wrap-around gowns that seemed less confusing and provided more coverage than our present styles. Like a tasty item at a local restaurant, good things usually are discontinued.

I'm waiting for the day a patient puts his legs through armholes like pants.

Fortunately, at the end of a day we can't bow and take credit for our patients' creativity, like fashion designers do at the end of a show. But some Paris designers might wish they could.

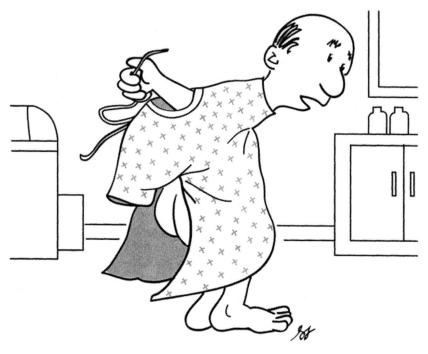

Nurse! This thing is the wrong size!

'Twas the Night before Christmas: Codes for the Holidays
Jamie L. Beeley, RN, BSN, MS, CRNA

'Twas the night before Christmas and in SICU
All the patients were stirring, the nurses were, too.
Some Levophed hung from an IMED with care
In hopes that a blood pressure soon would be there.
One patient was resting all snug in his bed
While visions—from Versed—danced in his head.
I, in my scrubs, with flow sheet in hand,
Had just settled down to chart the care plan.

Then from room 17 there arose such a clatter
We sprang from the station to see what was the matter.
Away to the beside we flew like a flash,
Saved the man there from falling, took restraints from the stash.
"Do you know where you are?" one nurse asked while tying;
"Of course! I'm in France in a jail and I'm dying!"

Then what to my wondering eyes should appear?
But a heart rate of 50, the alarm in my ear.
The patient's face paled, his skin became slick
And he said in a moment, I'm going to be sick!"
Someone found the Inapsine and injected a port,
Then ran for a basin, as if it were sport.
His heart rhythm quieted back to a sinus,
We soothed him and calmed him with old-fashioned kindness.

And then in a twinkling we heard from room 11
First a plea for assistance, then a swearing to heaven.
As I drew in my breath and was turning around,
Through the unit I hurried to respond to the sound.
"This one's having chest pain," the nurse said and then
She gave her some nitro, then morphine and when
She showed no relief from IV analgesia
Her breathing was failing: time to call anesthesia.

"Page Dr. Wilson, or May, or Banoub!
Get Dr. Epperson! She ought to be tubed!"
While the unit clerk paged them, the monitor showed
V-tach and low pressure with no pulse: "Call a code!"

More rapid than eagles, the code team they came.
The leader took charge and he called drugs by name:
"Now epi! Now Lido! Some bicarb and mag!
You shock and you chart it! You push meds! You bag!"
And so to the crash cart, the nurses we flew
With a handful of meds, and some dopamine, too.
From the head of the bed, the doc gave his call:
"Resume CPR!" So we worked one and all.
Then Doc said no more, but went straight to his work,
Intubated the patient, then turned with a jerk.
While placing his fingers to the side of her nose,
And giving a nod, hooked the vent to the hose.

The team placed an art-line and right triple-lumen.
And when they were through, she scarcely looked human:
Now an extraterrestrial hospital being,
For we'd track several waveforms and how much she's peeing.

When the patient was stable, the doc gave a whistle.
A progress note added as he wrote his epistle.
But I heard him exclaim, ere he strode out of sight,
"Merry Christmas to all! But no more codes for tonight!"
Reprinted from RN, ©1999; 62(12): 46 with permission from the author.

Fire Drill Protocol

During a recent fire drill, I was closing doors to patients' rooms. An 86-year-old patient was talking on the phone when I reached her room. As I started to shut her door, she asked, "What's that ringing noise?" *"Don't worry," I said. "We're just having a little fire drill."*

As I was leaving, I heard her say, "No, everything's just fine, dear. The hospital's on fire but a nice little nurse just came to lock me in my room."
From *This Won't Hurt a Bit!* Karyn Buxman, ©2000 LaMoine Press. Used with permission.

Passing Fads
Jane Bates

As a general principle, I believe we should tell the truth at all times, but there are occasions when honesty is not the best policy. It wasn't for the canny patient 30 years ago, at any rate. Of course, it is different now. Patients have a say in their treatment and thank goodness they do. But in my day, a little white lie about a certain bodily function was the only way to survive in hospital.

There was always the odd patient, who, when asked about their bowels, would give a blow-by-blow account of the life of their lower intestines. But most people, understandably, wanted to keep their toilet habits to themselves and would assert, unblushing, that they had their bowels open daily when they obviously had not, given the lack of exercise, bland diet and absence of privacy in the average ward.

What really terrified patients in those days was the ever-present threat of an enema. This was not a small warm package of glycerine solution. The enema of 30-something years ago was a very different animal. It was a two-nurse job, and not many things were in those days, which gave it some gravitas. It involved a laden trolley being wheeled up the ward in full view of the other patients, who, despite their evident *schaden-freude*, would avert their eyes respectfully.

There was something gung-ho about the procedure that scared the patients witless. The secret was 'high, hot and quite a lot', we were told, as the Heath Robinson construction of thick rubber tubing and funnels was assembled. Jugs of hot soapy water sat steaming ominously while I prayed that the patient would not look round.

There was an awful lot of tubing—yards of the stuff. I had apocryphal notions about the length of the intestines. Someone had told me that if you stretched them out straight, they would go from London to Newcastle—but even to my gullible eyes, the length of tubing seemed excessive. But a lot of it went somewhere. Before you could say 'syrup of figs' the patient would give a strangled gasp and in went the hot studs.

'Keep it in for 15 minutes,' the nurse would say, but no one ever managed more than five. For the nursing staff it was a matter of standing well back and quietly humming the closing bars of the *1812 Overture*. Then fetching the mop.

'Thank you nurse,' the patient would utter weakly, no doubt telling himself that there was a lot to be said for constipation. And also vowing that in the future, when sister gave him a penetrating stare and asked after his motions, the answer would be an unequivocal, 'absolutely perfect.'

Reprinted with permission from Nursing Standard, ©2002;16(22): 26. Edited from the original.

Kidney Confusion

After eight long months, a five-year-old boy finally got the call to come in for his kidney transplant. When the transplant coordinator went in to visit the boy and his parents, he was crying his eyes out, but wouldn't tell his parents why. Finally the coordinator sent the parents from the room so she could visit with him alone. When he could finally speak without crying, he said, "Is this kidney coming from a boy or a girl?" *"What difference would that make?" she asked encouragingly.* "Because... I don't want to have to sit down to pee!"

From *This Won't Hurt a Bit!* Karyn Buxman, ©2000 LaMoine Press. Used with permission.

More "Official Explanations" of Emergency Nursing
Kitty Gardner, BS, RN, CEN

1. Expect a bus load of patients to arrive when a staff meeting or a farewell party for a staff member is planned.

2. The day all the pillows that were in the emergency department the day before have disappeared and the laundry has no more is the day that all the patients with fractures and congestive heart failure come in. It is also the day the ice maker breaks.

3. *Always* believe it when someone drives up in a private car and runs in yelling, "The baby is coming!"

4. The patients in the most critical condition seem to arrive by car, not by ambulance. Sometimes they have driven themselves.

5. The first time you have sat down all day, the last patient has been discharged from the previous onslaught of arrivals, and all is quiet is the time administration walks through and says, "Oh, you are not busy today!" Someone on staff is usually reading the paper at this time and the ED physician's feet are propped up on the counter.

Reprinted from Journal of Emergency Nursing, ©1992;18(3): 195 with permission from The Emergency Nurses Association.

Hold the Mayo
Hazel Lavender, RN

As a home health nurse, I recently visited a patient whose dressing supplies were almost nil. After thoroughly washing my hands, I noticed that there was no trash bag available, so I pulled one out of my nursing bag. Then I needed solution and gauze to cleanse the patient's wounds, so out they came, followed by sterile dry dressings to cover the wounds. Finally, I needed tape. As I searched for it in what must have seemed like a bottomless bag, the patient queried, "Do you have a ham and cheese sandwich in there, too?"

Reprinted with permission from RN, ©2004;67(8): 12. RN is a copyrighted publication of Advanstar Communications Inc. All rights reserved.

Medical Mishaps
Kathy A. Brink, RN

Sometimes The Truth Is More Amusing Than Fiction...

- A man comes into the ER and yells, "My wife's going to have her baby in the cab! The ER physician grabs his stuff, rushes out to the cab, lifts the lady's dress, and begins to take off her underwear. Suddenly he notices that there are several cabs, and he's in the wrong one.

- A nurse at the beginning of the shift places her stethoscope on an elderly and slightly deaf female patient's anterior chest wall. "Big breaths," instructed the nurse. "Yes, they used to be," remarked the patient.

- One day I had to be the bearer of bad news when I told a wife that her husband had died of a massive myocardial infarct. Not more than five minutes later, I heard her reporting to the rest of the family that he had died of a "massive internal fart."

- I was performing a complete physical, including the visual acuity test. I placed the patient twenty feet from the chart and began, "Cover your right eye with your hand." He read the 20/20 line perfectly. "Now your left." Again, a flawless read. "Now both," I requested. There was silence. He couldn't' even read the large E on the top line. I turned and discovered that he had done exactly what I had asked; he was standing there with both his eyes covered. I was laughing too hard to finish the exam.

- A nurses' aide was helping a patient into the bathroom when the patient exclaimed, "You're not coming in here with me. This is only a one-seater!"

- During a patient's two week follow-up appointment with his cardiologist, he informed his doctor that he was having trouble with one of his medications. "Which one?", asked the doctor. "The patch." The nurse told me to put on a new one every six hours and now I'm running out of places to put it!" The doctor had him quickly undress and discovered what he hoped he wouldn't' see....Yes, the man had over fifty patches on his body! Now the instructions include removal of the old patch before applying a new one.

- While acquainting myself with a new elderly patient, I asked, "How long have you been bedridden?" After a look of complete confusion she answered, "Why not for about twenty years-when my husband was alive."

And of course, the best is saved for last...

- A nurse caring for a woman from Kentucky asked, "So how's your breakfast this morning?" "It's very good, except for the Kentucky Jelly. I can't seem to get used to the taste," the patient replied. The nurse asked to see the jelly and the woman produced a foil packet labeled... "KY Jelly."

Reprinted with permission. Retrieved December 6, 2004 from Medi-Smart, Inc. Web site www.medi-smart.com

Pre-op Instructions as Our Patients Hear Them
March Warn, RN

Diet and NPO Instructions

Surgery can be a stressful experience. It is necessary that you prepare your body for this experience by providing the necessary fuel. We suggest that on the way into the hospital you stop and have a hearty breakfast. Steak and eggs, hash browns, biscuits and gravy, at least two cups of coffee, and a large orange juice should see you through your surgical experience.

If your child is scheduled for surgery, he or she will likely be cranky on the trip into the hospital. Stop at a convenience store and get a large Coke and a Twinkie to settle your child down.

Clothing/Makeup

Since you will be seen by a large number of people while in our waiting room, we suggest that you dress up in your finest clothing and jewelry. Do not forget to apply a full coat of makeup, since you probably look sickly without it. If you are scheduled for a gynecologic procedure, be sure to wear pantyhose and a girdle. Several thicknesses of a bright nail polish will impress the surgical team with your fashion sense. And, so the admitting nurse will have no questions about your ability to pay your bill, wear every piece of jewelry you own.

Children scheduled for surgery should be dressed in their finest clothing, preferably bought just for this occasion, especially if they are going to have a tonsillectomy or tooth extraction. Large, heavy shoes with hard, sharp soles will keep their feet warm in the recovery room. Be sure to tie the laces in complex knots so your child cannot remove them easily.

Arrival Time

We will give you a time when you should arrive at the hospital. However, because hospitals, like doctors' offices, always run late, it is best to arrive at least 2 hours after that appointment time. This will prevent a long, boring session in our waiting room.

Diagnostic Test Results

If your referring doctor has given you copies of any diagnostic tests he or she may have performed at their office, do not bring these with you. We have a fax machine, and our secretary really enjoys calling doctors' offices to have test results faxed over. (We don't think she ever gets any good mail at home, so this is very exciting for her.)

Home Medications

If you are taking any medications at home on a regular basis, we would like to know about them. It is not necessary for you to know the name or your dose of these medications. Just a general description will do. For instance, you can tell us that you take half a pink football, two plain round white pills and a speckled capsule at breakfast, and the rest of the pink football at bedtime. We will know exactly what you are taking because we are trained professionals and can identify all medications by their color and shape.

Past Medical/Surgical History

It is not necessary for you to know detailed information about your medical history. Just tell us you have had "stomach trouble" or that sometime in the past, a doctor once said you had "a funny heart sound." And, if you have ever had relatives whose surgery was canceled because they ran very high fevers after they were given anesthesia, do not tell us or we might cancel your surgery and you will have taken a day off from work for nothing. We do not need to know that you bleed for several hours any time you cut yourself shaving, or that you bruise easily. All surgical patients are going to bleed anyway.

You need not tell us about your surgical history. If you can't remember whether you have had your gallbladder, appendix, uterus, or ovaries removed, do not worry. One of our favorite OR games is called "guess the surgery." After you are asleep, we try to guess which organs you have had removed by interpreting the scars on your body. And if you can't remember which side your hernia, breast lump, lipoma, or varicose vein is on, we will simply make an educated guess. We have a 50-50 chance of being correct.

Transportation

You will likely be given lots of narcotic and anesthetic agents while you are in surgery. After surgery, you may be drowsy or have diminished reflexes. You would not want any of your family members or friends to see you in this condition, so drive yourself to the hospital and do not make arrangements for anyone to drive you home. After all, once you get out of the city, it is a straight shot up the interstate to your house.

Reprinted with permission from Journal of Nursing Jocularity, ©1996; 6(4): 22-23. Edited from the original.

Pot Luck
Jane Bates

Isn't it a marvel, the diversity of containers people transport their urine samples in? We all know the story of the man who used a whisky bottle as a wee receptacle, label still attached 'finest single malt, 70 per cent proof,' who had it stolen from his bag en route to hospital.

Doesn't bear thinking about, does it? Except the thief probably went off whisky. Probably renounced his life of crime as well, and is now leading an exemplary life in Hemel Hempstead.

Which of us, as nurses, has not fallen victim to the medicine bottle with the impossible-to-shift childproof lid? Or been fooled by urine in the jam jar into thinking the patient is diabetic? Spice and pickle jars, cola and milk bottles, they've all been used to accommodate the requisite sample. And you can tell a lot about a patient by their choice of pot.

The 'professional' patient uses a proper specimen container and, what's more, labels it. The generous soul fills it to the brim so that it splatters all over you as you open it. You know, you just know, that it's leaked all over the inside of their handbag. And there's the parsimonious patient who provides you with a dribble ('I know it's not much, it's all I could manage'), usually in a tall, narrow-necked bottle, so that it is well-nigh impossible to get the testing stick into the urine.

I was once presented with a sample in a Tupperware box—they are watertight—which I was instructed to wash out and hand back, no doubt so that the gentleman could use it for his packed lunch the next day. But my favorite wee-container story has to be from a midwife I worked with in London's East End. A mother-to-be always brought her urine specimen to the clinic in a cracked, chipped old china cup (no lid), full to the brim and with the contents sloshing all over her feet. This was always washed and duly returned to her for the next appointment.

When my colleague went to pay her first postnatal visit, the grateful mother handed her some tea—and the midwife recognized the cup immediately. To her great credit, she downed the lot without batting an eyelid.

Reprinted with permission from Nursing Standard, ©2001; 16(12): 23.

How High is Too High?
Robert S. Kirk, RN

A patient of mine on the dementia/Alzheimer's unit is a very withdrawn woman who barely eats, rarely participates in activities, and routinely answers questions with a one-word response. Until one day recently, that is.

To assess for peripheral circulation, I knelt by her chair, loosened her shoe, and felt for a pedal pulse. Unable to find one easily, I tried for the popliteal pulse behind her knee. Imagine my surprise when she looked directly at me and asked, "Just how high are you planning to go?"

Even Nurses Have to Laugh
Sheila Rogers, RN

Working in a hospital emergency room has its moments—most of them serious, a few quite the opposite. Among the few, these are some that have brightened my day.

This one patient had accidentally ingested antifreeze stored in a grape juice bottle that somehow had found its way into the refrigerator. Only a few swallows were required for him to realize that this wasn't grape juice at all.

The standard treatment for ethylene glycol poisoning, which is what the antifreeze had given him, is intravenous alcohol. As I was explaining this to the man, he politely asked for some Tylenol. I was a bit puzzled because he had yet to complain of any pain. He then explained that he just wanted to get the jump on his impending hangover.

Another incident involved a child who had decided to play with Bondo, the epoxy-like resin used for sealing holes in cars. When the medics brought the child in, along with the can of Bondo, the boy had it all over his hands and face. The fumes from the can were so powerful that the ambulance driver made the entire trip holding the can out of the window. Though the boy suffered no serious effects, it just goes to show that kids can and will get into anything.

I remember another little fellow coming in with a mild swelling in his upper lip after he had tasted a flower he'd come upon while walking in a field with his parents. Being "city folks," they were not sure if this plant has poisoned their son. The doctor was trying to draw a picture of this "poison," which the family had brought with them.

Finally, it was up to me, a country girl, to walk up and identify the wicked weed as a common clover, found in any pasture. It was something I had enjoyed many times as a child because of its sweet taste. The patient was quickly released with a diagnosis of a simple allergic reaction instead of poisoning.

I once triaged a woman who had Alzheimer's disease. I began by checking her level of orientation with the usual list of questions. When asked her name, she gave it, no problem. When asked where she was, she quickly replied, "At the hospital." When asked the name of the President of the United States, she just couldn't come up with the answer. After she had thought awhile, she finally said, "I can't remember his name, but he's that young man who makes his wife do all the work." When I asked if she was referring to President Clinton, she just gave me a big wink and a smile.

Another nurse told me about a man who came to the emergency department stating that he had a cut finger. He was pale, sweaty, and just about to pass out. Because his hand was in a large basin partially filled with blood, the nurse rushed him to a treatment room, thinking the guy must have severed an artery. As it turned out, only two stitches were required to repair his wound. The blood belonged to the poor pig he had been trying to castrate.

Then there was a teenager in an auto accident who had not been wearing a seat belt and had struck his head on the windshield. Awake but confused, he continually asked, "Why was everyone there speaking Chinese?" After I had answered "I don't know" for the 30th time, I dismissed the question as part of his concussion. Just then a police officer arrived to question the boy. In the process, the officer happened to mention that this case was very difficult because the other vehicle contained five non-English-speaking adults from China.

I still think of the little boy who had broken his arm and was waiting for x-rays. His cart happened to be parked under a large silver wall panel whose only purpose was to provide access to some electric wires. The little chap was crying, so I stopped to see if I could offer some comfort. It seems the thought of the x-rays wasn't what bothered him; his crying had to do with the "dead bodies" behind that silver panel. After I opened the panel and showed him the wires, his tears dried up in a hurry.

What a shame that all emergency cases can't be solved so easily!

Reprinted with permission from The Saturday Evening Post Magazine, ©January/February 2000, Saturday Evening Post Society.

You're the Top

Why Are Nurses Considered Angels?

- Is it because their shoes allow them to seemingly float from room to room?
- Is it because of their ability to predict outcomes even if you do not follow their instructions?
- Is it because they are there in your hour of need?
- Is it because they have that angelic touch?
- Is it because they can tell everyone where to go with authority?

Despite these qualities, it only takes a member of their family to bring them down to earth.

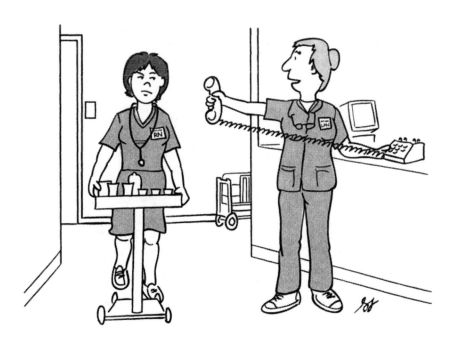

Your husband wants to know where his socks are.

Treat Your Nurse Right

When you're hospitalized, it pays to be nice to your nurse, even when you're feeling miserable. A bossy businessman learned the hard way after ordering his nurses around as if they were his employees. But the head nurse stood up to him.

One morning she entered his room and announced, "I have to take your temperature."

After complaining for several minutes, he finally settled down, crossed his arms and opened his mouth.

"No, I'm sorry," the nurse stated, "but for this reading, I can't use an oral thermometer." This started another round of complaining, but eventually he rolled over and bared his bottom.

After feeling the nurse insert the thermometer, he heard her announce, "I have to get something. Now you stay just like that until I get back!"

She left the door to his room open on her way out, and he cursed under his breath as he heard people walking past his door laughing. After almost an hour, the man's doctor came into the room.

"What's going on here?" asked the doctor.

Angrily, the man answers, "What's the matter, Doc? Haven't you ever seen someone having their temperature taken?"

"Yes," said the doctor. "But never with a carnation."

Reprinted with permission. Retrieved December 6, 2004 from Medi-Smart, Inc. Web site: www.medi-smart.com

It's Hard to Live with a Nurse Because...

- When you forget to flush the toilet, you get a complete analysis with a plan on how to correct any noted problems.

- Thanksgiving dinner comes in pre-cut small pieces because she doesn't want to have to perform the Heimlich maneuver and be reminded of work on the only holiday she's had off in years.

- You've been awakened from a dead sleep in the middle of the night to find her shaking you because your breathing patterns were a little too close to a Cheyne-Stokes rhythm.

Reprinted with permission. Retrieved June 27, 2005 from www.nursinghumor.com

True Life: The World According to a Practice Nurse
Sarah Johnson

Crucial matters such as who spends half an hour under the spare bed trying to drag the cat out as we leave for a holiday or whose turn it is to sit and systematically pick the slugs off the hostas which now resemble shredded cabbage, do spark off occasional rucks.

Still, I think I realised the mashed potato missiles would be aimed at me when I tried venting my frustration over Tuesday supper—bemoaning my regular targets, the patients who waste my time at the surgery.

I was subjected to a barrage of outrage from my family. The problem it would seem, is that I (Mrs. Practicality) do not live in the real world.

It is much worse for the other patients waiting behind the moaning time-wasters than it is for me, my husband assured me.

I looked incredulous.

'Imagine how it feels,' he said. 'For a person who rarely goes to the doctors—say about once every eight years—who first has to circumnavigate the most intimidating person in the world.' (I hazard a guess—although I may be wrong—this is the receptionist!)

He continues: 'Then they are penalised for their lack of attendance by being offered an appointment with a doctor who may be capable of a diagnosis three weeks on Thursday. Or, alternatively, they can have an appointment with the duff doctor which is about as good as giving themselves two paracetamol and consulting the goods manager at work.' Having vented his frustration my husband slumped back in his chair and relaxed.

I was about to clarify some of the not too subtle points when my teenage daughter Holly summed up the problem for me.

'The thing is Mum you just know that there's no one that's, like, as ill as you are. You can tell by looking at them they're OK. I sit there in that waiting room wasting away because of all those people who use it as a day out.'

'Mmm, another rounded teenage argument,' I thought.

But my mind was still ten minutes previous. 'Which duff doctor?' I spurted.

'The one that always has to get his drug book out,' said my husband.

'Oh honestly, I do that.'

So anyway, I have come up with the solution to patient waiting room frustration. We as a Service provider need to be more open to cosmetic improvements. But how should we go about it? I mean this could be taken to extremes, we could use feng-shui in the surgery. This could be done in much the same way as you would your own home.

Yes the patients could all end up facing the disabled toilet but spiritually they may feel lifted. One could place strategic plants in areas that do not lend themselves to positive vibes. Speaking to a receptionist through a small forest could be challenging but none-the-less may create a perfect karma.

A less radical approach may be to invest in an airport lounge environment. Piped music and a coffee machine along with small melodic announcements informing the waiting public just exactly how late the doctor is running, could go some way to reduce the frustration patients feel when 25 minutes has elapsed and the previous patient has still not emerged from the doctor's room.

We could also employ in-house pharmacists to reduce doctor consultation time. It could run something like this.

GP: 'Well Mr. Jones it would appear that you are suffering from angina and may need some medication, please take this yellow card and make your way along to room 17 where the pharmacist will advise you of the current drugs available.'

Oh all right, perhaps not that, but we could meet the patients half way with very little added expense. Wheel a telly into the waiting room and stick on Eastenders!

Reprinted with permission from Practice Nurse, ©2001; 22(9): 62.

The Nurse
Bob McKenty

Armed with thermometer, needle and grin,
She's determined *somehow* to get under my skin.

Reprinted with permission from American Journal of Nursing, ©1975; 75(5): 914.

This Time I Mean It
Deb Gauldin, RN, PMS

Contractions are like waves ... coming and going, coming and going. In a given day, my moods cycle up, then down, up and down, coming and going. And over the years, an even larger life pattern has emerged. It is the pattern of realizing I am overwhelmed and overstressed, cutting back, swearing I will never let this happen again, then in no time finding myself coming and going and going and going!

With firm resolve, I vowed that this year I would be extremely discerning about what tasks I volunteered to do. I practiced pausing and calming, reciting my new mantra: "Let me give that some consideration and I'll get back to you."

The phone rang. It was the school librarian. "Mrs. Gauldin," she said. "Would you be kind enough to come into the grade school on Thursday and help with AIDS?" I paused, recited my well-rehearsed mantra and proceeded to step 2 of my new approach.

Hanging up, I turned off the radio, sat down at the kitchen table, lit a candle, and began a combination of deep breaths and progressive relaxation. I would agree *only* if I determined an opportunity to be meaningful.

AIDS hmmm. Who better to come in to speak and sing about AIDS? I even knew a song about the AIDS quilt. Yes, yes. This was meaningful.

When I returned Mrs. Spanogle's call, she appreciatively scheduled me from noon to 3:00 PM. Now I love health education, but there was no way I had enough songs about AIDS to fill three hours!

Mrs. Spanogle emphatically continued, "We sure don't want the children burning themselves."

Burning themselves? What?

"You know," she went on. "While dripping hot candle wax on the eggs."

Eggs? Eggs! I thought she had said AIDS! She wanted me to help the kids make Ukrainian Easter eggs! Thoughts swirling, I could barely choke out a trembling response. Eggs? Eggs aren't meaningful!

I have no idea what she thought of that day and, as you might have guessed, I spent the following Thursday afternoon like the Easter Bunny, meaningfully coloring eggs! Perhaps more like the Energizer® Bunny. That is, I keep on going and going and going.

What's In a Name
Amy Y. Young, BS, MLS

Language plays a major role in everyday communication and supposedly separates us from other species and makes us superior to them. Words are fascinating and the local phone book will affirm your belief that everyday words can play a major part in the nursing profession. Think positive, your name can say a whole lot about you.

Admissions Nurse	Nurse Dorman
Army Nurse	Nurse March
Camp Nurse	Nurse Summers
	Nurse Camp
Cardiology	Nurse Hart

Community Health Nurse	Nurse Well
Corrections Nurse	Nurse Jailer
ENT	Nurse Knowles
Emergency Room Nurse	Nurse Blood
	Nurse Gore
Endocrinology	Nurse Glans
Flight Nurse	Nurse Flyer
Gerontology Nurse	Nurse Olde
Grant Applicant	Nurse Grant
Home Health Nurse	Nurse Holmes
	Nurse Homer
Hospice Nurse	Nurse Terminello
Hospital Nurse	Nurse Ward
Industrial Nurse	Nurse Machine
Infertility Clinic	Nurse Egg
Labor & Delivery	Nurse Pushkin
Management	Nurse Boss
Military Nurse	Nurse Warr
Neonatal Nurse	Nurse Young
	Nurse Bambino
Night Shift	Nurse Knight
Nurse Administrator	Nurse Planz
Nurse Anesthetist	Nurse Sleep
Nurse Educator	Nurse Edu-Daly
Nurse Midwife	Nurse Birthwright
	Nurse Bourne
Nurse Supervisor	Nurse Super
	Nurse Bossey
Nurse Theorist	Nurse Thierry
Nurse Recruiter	Nurse Hunter
Nurses' Aide	Nurse Aide
Nursing Home	Nurse Elder
Obstetrics & Gynecology	Nurse Stirrup
Occupational Health	Nurse Hazard
Oncology	Nurse Metasin
Ophthalmology	Nurse Vision
Orthopedics	Nurse Bone
Pediatrics	Nurse Childe
Plastic Surgery	Nurse Tuck
Preventive Health	Nurse Populus
Proctology	Nurse Bower
Psychiatric	Nurse Kranks
	Nurse Looney

Public Health	Nurse Publico
	Nurse Globus
Radiology	Nurse Gama
Rehabilitation	Nurse Strong
Retiring Nurse	Nurse Exito
School Nurse	Nurse Schooler
Ship Nurse	Nurse Shippe
Staff Nurse	Nurse Officer
Substance Abuse	Nurse Druga
	Nurse Narker
	Nurse Boos
Triage Nurse	Nurse Crisci
	Nurse Crisses
Surgical Nurse	Nurse Cutter
Trauma	Nurse Strain
Urologic	Nurse Ureta
Vacationing Nurse	Nurse Holliday
Visiting Nurse	Nurse Visintin

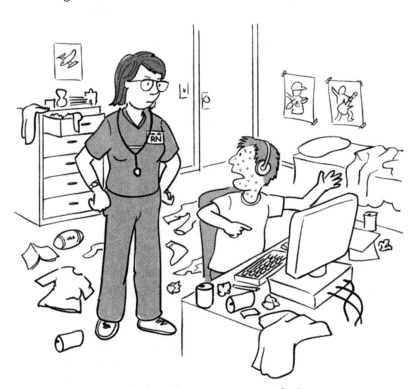

Mom, I looked up all my symptoms on the internet
and I think I should be dead!

Nurses Do It Better

Claire Ligeikis-Clayton, RN

My neighbor's 3-year-old son got a splinter in his foot while he was playing at our summer cottage. After trying unsuccessfully to remove it, his mother told him, "We'll go see Uncle Don. He's a surgeon—he'll get the splinter out."

"I don't want Uncle Don to take it out," the little boy insisted. "I want a real doctor to take out my splinter. I want a nurse!"

We Are a Funny Lot

Ged Cowin RN, BEd

My husband works on a hospital ward. He is not a nurse but works closely with them and the other night he announced that nurses are a funny lot.

I asked him why and he said that he has noticed three outstanding things about nurses:
- We understate catastrophe,
- We laugh at the most bizarre moments, and,
- We eat and walk incredibly fast.

I pointed out that was actually four things, but that's beside the point.

I thought about it for a minute and whilst I wouldn't have pulled these things out as the most important attributes of a nurse, I concluded that in a way he is right.

I thought of a cardiac arrest situation. There is a flurry of activity, exhausted nurses doing basic life support, drugs flying over a crowd of heads, shouting, rushing and at the end when the patient's heart has resumed normal activity—as well as your own—you say to the patient: "It's okay, Mr. Jones, you've had a bit of a turn."

A bit of turn! Now we don't even say a big turn, or a turn to be afraid of. No, it's a bit of turn.

My mum is 71 years old. She rang me distressed the other day because she had fallen over and hurt her ankle.

Being the nurse of the family, I raced around, did the examinations—declared her fit, albeit bruised, and assured her she was still for this earth for quite a bit longer.

Next, I sat down at her telephone and rang the family—all eight brothers and sisters—and pronounced to all that mum 'had a fall'.

When I'd finished, mum looked at me and said: 'so, had a fall eh? I've crossed over.'

"What do you mean?' I asked.

She said that there is a magical age when you stop simply falling over and start 'having falls.'

I chuckled a bit at this, though she was not amused.

We, as nurses, especially, do tend to imply an awful lot in a simple phrase.

Once someone has 'had a fall', suddenly they are not trusted to be able to get up again and it implies the need of support and looking after.

If I told people I'd fallen over they would probably laugh and assume I'd had too much to drink. I tell them Mum's 'had a fall' and they all nod in concern.

We are often masters of understatement and tend to play things down. Maybe because we want to keep things calm, ourselves included. We don't want to alarm or cause concern or make a situation worse.

I know my children need to have gaping wounds pumping blood from arteries before I'll admit to them that 'putting up with it' won't actually help.

And as for laughing, well how else do we cope? I remember as a student nurse doing a soap and water enema with a partner in crime. I know, we don't do them anymore.

We had a bucket, a hose, a funnel, plastic sheeting, plastic aprons, gloves and gumboots—and we had soap and water from one end of the room to the other. We were wading in it—good stuff and all.

And we got the giggles something shocking, so much so we had to cover the patient up and leave to let it all out.

That poor patient, I often think of her. We just couldn't help it.

We've all got stories like that. And as for eating and walking fast, that comes with the job.

There's no real moral or point to make of all this, just that I guess we are a funny lot.

Reprinted with permission from Australian Nursing Journal, ©Dec 2001/Jan 2002; 9(6): 48.

Achy Breaky Neck
Maynard Good Stoddard

Now that we have dismissed as ridiculous the subject of my trifling with the truth, I said to my dear wife, Lois, "how about discussing the episodes in which you have unquestionably tried to kill me?"

"I've never tried to do you in," she protested, chuckling over what must have been remembrance of one of the episodes.

It could have been the one in which I had no more than mounted the seat of my big red 11-horse Murray mower than she yelled above the roar of its mighty engine, "While you're at it, how about mowing under the pine trees while I hold the branches back?"

At this point, I should have remembered how she had promised to hold the stepladder while I strung lights on the blue spruce we were decorating for our first (and last) outdoor Christmas tree. No sooner had I arrived on the most treacherous step on the ladder than over it went, leaving me draped across the barbed wire fence. The puncture wounds would leave my frontal area looking like a cribbage board for the next two weeks.

Upon inquiry, it seems that she had let go of the ladder because the next string of lights was tangled and she knew I'd be mad if she handed it up to me before straightening it out.

"Better mad than dead," I explained, my gentle breeding being the only deterrent to straightening her out.

So now she would be holding the branches back while I mowed under the pine trees. Common sense being not all that common, I fell for it.

Give the dear girl credit; not until way along on branch number two did she let it go, just as I was approaching. (Her glove had come off, she explained with a straight face.) The released limb having knocked me off the mower, dear wife heroically flung herself across the vacated seat and directed the vehicle through the branches of the adjoining tree until it slammed to a stop against the trunk.

Only after shutting off the engine and walking twice around the mower did she come over to where I was lying and say, "Don't worry; it's not hurt a bit."

Perhaps you remember when she assigned me the task of painting the outside trim on the window frame where she couldn't reach and thoughtfully had erected a scaffold for my convenience. She contrived the scaffold by suspending a board between a potato crate and a stack of bricks, with the rotten side of the board cleverly turned under. I no more than dipped my brush into this gallon bucket of black paint than the board gave way, causing me to paint a stripe the full length of the window on my way down. What the bucket of paint did to my Greek-god torso below the waist remains unrecorded.

I once went three full days without bleeding a drop. Thinking that this might be bad for my circulatory system, my concerned wife began hanging cast-iron pots from the ceiling, filling them with potting soil, adding a sprig of hollyhock, and calling the result macramé. What I called these booby traps has also gone unrecorded. Standing a mere 5'5" in high heels, she cleared the devices nicely, whereas they caught me just above the eyebrows. As a result, the well-shaped head I once prided myself on soon assumed the contour of a Hubbard squash.

Installation of the pipe for our Ben Franklin wood-burning stove provided yet another opportunity for my dear wife to collect on my life insurance policy and head for Rio and a handkissing Latin vulture. Her part in this looming disaster was to support the stovepipe with the broom while I, from the convenience of a stepstool, directed the five lengths of pipe into the chimney hole.

Why a healthy woman's arms would give out, as she claimed, after only 15 minutes has never been cleared up to my satisfaction. What I do know is, when the stove lengths parted company, the one directly above my head relieved me of my already shaky stance on the footstool, and had it not been for the layer of soot now covering the floor, that might well have been all she wrote right there.

This brings us to the episode that will likely go down in the family annals as The Day Dear Wife Removed the Ladder. Hoping to reduce, or by some miracle completely stop the leak, I had been talked into scaling the ladder to tar the metal roof over our glassed-in front porch. Because of the pitch of the roof, however, no sooner had I inched my way to the top of the incline than I began sliding back. Looking around to make sure my feet would hit the ladder ... no ladder!

Luckily, by now, the bucket of tar had tipped over, coating my underside and slowing my descent, thereby providing several more seconds for my life to pass before me. Not until my remains had been discovered behind the spirea would I learn that dear wife had borrowed the ladder "while I was up there" to pull ivy off the siding. She became upset for having to explain it three different times, my upturned ear being filled with tar at the time.

I still have nightmares from my attempt to get into the exercise thing by doing a few leisurely situps. Discovering that I was unable to sit up without hooking my toes under something, I went into the kitchen to hook them under the electric range. Along about number three trying for four, my bride of 57 summers (I don't count the winters, because of those ski-type pajamas) came in from her annual chore of mopping the back porch.

"Oh, good heavens!" she cried, dropping her mop and bucket of suds and straddling my stomach, from which position she began hammering on my chest.

"What-in-the-blue-blazes-do-you-think-you-are-doing?" I sputtered.

"EPA," she explained, obviously pleased that she had revived me to the point where I could talk.

"It's CPR," I moaned. "EPA is the Environmental Protection Agency, for Pete's sake!"

"Whatever... it has saved your life."

"You came closer to killing me," I said, dumping her off, removing the mop handle from my forehead, and wringing the still-hot suds out of my sweatshirt. "I was only attempting a few sit-ups."

"And you've probably got the stove all out of kilter," she said by way of apology.

Finally (and I'm sure you are more than ready—I know I am), I call your attention to the birdbath experience. It happened after my dear wife complained, "The birdbath is full of water." You are probably thinking a woman has to be hard up for complaints to reach this level. But no, the problem was that the birds had never so much as dipped a toe in this concrete lavatory to test the water. That's why we were using it as a feeding station.

Now, I had been asked to leave the refuge of my typewriter, gird up my loins, and tip up this 80- or 90-pound bowl to let the water drain. Having failed to gird my loins high enough, however, the thing got away from me, and all 150 pounds landed on my best foot, the one without the black toenail from another incident we won't go into. Only a determined will to live got me back into the house.

"What happened to you?" asked you-know-who.

"The birdbath fell on my foot," I whined. "Oh," she said, resuming her hanging of another macrame device in my new route to the bathroom. "I thought maybe you'd been hurt."

That's the trouble with being married to a nurse. I could come in with my head hanging from a single neck cord, and she'd say, "I can remember a man coming into Emergency carrying his head under his arm...take a couple of aspirin and forget it."

©Maynard Good Stoddard. Reprinted with permission from The Saturday Evening Post magazine, ©1994; 266(5): 52-53.

Bubbles

Robyn Maxwell, RN, BSN

Have you ever had one of those "horrible days" in your nursing career, where everything seems to go wrong? Let me share mine with you...

I am a nurse manager at a large hospital in Tulsa. Here is the gist of how the day started. Just imagine a peak census on the unit, a snow day when half the staff could not make it in (including the unit secretary), and a hospital-wide skin prevalence study. I was brushing up on my clinical secretary skills and trying to enter orders. Then I had the opportunity to see every patient's skin from head to toe on my unit. The staff seemed to be laughing to themselves watching the "manager try to do it." All the while I still had to do my "manager job" and help my skeleton crew. There would be no time for lunch or even coffee today. I couldn't wait for that day to be over.

I just kept promising myself that when I got home I would relax, have a glass of wine, and take a bubble bath with no interruptions from my work or family. When I arrive home I formally advised my husband and 9-year-old daughter that, "Mommy had a terrible day at work," and would need some rest and relaxation time for a few minutes. I ran my bath, filled it with very hot water and as many bubbles as I possibly could. I had just got in the water, and then it happened…

I suddenly heard the sound of pounding feet running down the hall towards my bathroom door. I wondered, don't they know it is my time? The door slammed open and there stood my husband with a dusky complexion and a look of panic on his face. OK, so is he having a heart attack or what? I wondered. He couldn't speak.

"Are you having a heart attack, or are you choking?" The good news was that he was not having a heart attack, the bad news was that he was choking. Now keep in mind that I just recently grumbled through a whole day of CPR. I had let my certification expire so I had to sit though the whole 8 hour class again. I had also just finished renewing my ACLS too, so I felt well equipped to handle the situation. I stayed very calm; I was just not too pleased that I was not dressed for this homespun crisis. Yes, you have the picture. I was nude with only bubbles on. No time for a robe when your husband is choking. Time is of the essence! So I went through all the Heimlich maneuver, and my husband still was not breathing. My daughter walked in and to her surprise, saw Mommy standing in the bathroom in her birthday suit with her arms wrapped around Daddy.

I really didn't appreciate the visual in the mirror. I have gained a "little" weight since I became a nurse. Well, it was too late to contemplate a tummy tuck. My husband really needed me, but I wish if he had to be choking that I could at least be dressed for the occasion. Now what would I do if I have to start CPR and have my daughter call 911? When would be a good time to get dressed—before or after the ambulance came? I didn't remember covering that in CPR class.

It seemed like an eternity. This time I planned to do the "extreme" Heimlich maneuver. He may vomit everywhere, but maybe he would live. Yea, it worked! The father of my child, the husband that I adore and love, is going to live. As for the clothing quandary, I guess we'll never know.

My husband now adores me like when we were first married. He calls me 20 times a day to say thank you and tell me how much he loves me. Now that my daughter understands what happened, she also thinks Mommy is the greatest and she also calls me at work to say thank you for saving her Daddy's life. I am going to enjoy all this adoring attention while it lasts. Now where did I put that bottle of bubble bath…

Reprinted with permission from Oklahoma Nurse, ©2005; 50(1): 23.

Can You Hear Me Now?
Agnes H. Goldsmith, RN

As Thanksgiving opens up the holiday season, we look forward to more great food, festive parties, and spending time with friends and family. Amid the festivities, let us not forget the meaning that our families bring to us. They are the source of our greatest joys—and also the source of the most monumental frustrations known to man or woman. I say that, of course, in the most loving way.

During every holiday dinner, there are always a zillion conversations going on at the dinner table at one time. Somehow they seem louder and more passionate at my in-laws' table than at any other in the universe. Have you ever sat at a big holiday family gathering feeling you were in a hotter seat than the turkey in the roaster? Perhaps some of you can relate.

"Did you remember to bring it?" "Yes, Mom," I answer in the doorway, holding up the sweet potato casserole. "No, not that. The blood pressure cuff," she says. Hoping she'd forgotten, I reluctantly answer, "yes." I know my role as a nurse—the family's "consigliatore" for dispensing knowledgeable but unheeded healthcare advice.

Who is the first one family members ask about healthcare issues and the absolute last one on earth they listen to? The nurse in the family—who else? For some mysterious reason mom thinks the cashier at the grocery store, her hairdresser, and even the stranger in the cold and allergy medication aisle seem to dispense better healthcare information than we humble nurses. Do you ever want to say out loud what you only dare think to yourself—"If you've already decided to take the deli lady's advice, why are you asking me?"

Aunt Matilda spots me right off the bat. Before I catch my breath from her bear hug she pulls me by the arm and says, "Come with me for a second; let me show you this rash." Waving "hi" to everyone, off we go to check out the rash. "Aunt Matilda, this looks like hives, but I'm not a dermatologist; let me refer you to Dr. Stein." "So who is this doctor?" she asks. "Please, Aunt Matilda, just make an appointment." She says, "I thought you were a nurse; why can't you just give me a sample cream?" "I can't."

Oh, have I mentioned the noise level? "Uncle Morris has high blood pressure, just check it. It will only take you a second," shouts Mom into my ear. Blood pressure cuff and stethoscope in hand, I sit next to Uncle Morris. "I feel great. There's nothing wrong with me." When I note a BP of 160/90 I say to Uncle Morris, "When was the last time you had a checkup?" I'm fine, I don't need to see a doctor. I took my blood pressure medication last month and now I'm fine," he says. "Please, Uncle Morris, go see your doctor and take your medicine like you're supposed to. This is not a one-time prescription. It's really important to take it every day."

Sitting at the table, checking the desserts with my dad, I ask, "How are you doing with your diabetes?" "No problem," he says. "I haven't eaten sausages in months. No fat." "No, Dad," I say, "high fat increases your cholesterol level; high blood sugar levels are what you worry about in diabetes." "Fat, sugar, what's the difference, I can't even enjoy my food anymore." "Please watch what you're eating." "Look," he says, talking over me, "I've been a diabetic for 50 years and I've managed fine. Stop preaching to me." "Dad, please don't eat the pies — stick with the fruit."

Oh, did I mention the noise level? Industrial strength earplugs might bring the noise down to a tolerable, loud fire drill. Naturally at holiday time all the kids know the rules are out the window. "Michael, don't run with the knife, please bring it to me." "Slow down, guys, or somebody's going to get hurt." "Didn't you hear Aunt Jennifer? No ball-playing in the house." "Sammy, let your sister play." "Mom, Jason's jumping on the bed!" I just sit there taking it all in, enjoying the moment—and waiting knowingly for the inevitable closing bell. And there it is, an eerie split-second of silence, then the blood-curdling cry. Someone got hurt—my call to duty.

"Where's Aunt Aggie, go get Aunt Aggie!" "I'm right here," I say as I brush past all but one miraculously silent kid. "What happened?" I ask. Jason (the injured party), holding up his hand, yells between his sobs, "Michael broke my hand and I didn't even do anything! He just slammed the door on my hand!" A quick assessment as we head to the kitchen for the ice: No bleeding, no bruising yet, a little swelling beginning, fingernail beds have good blanching, fingers moving, no concentrated localized pain. Nursing diagnosis—moderately bruised hand and seriously bruised ego. Plan of care—ice for the hand, ice cream, and lots of one-on-one TLC for the ego.

Everyone returns to conversing—or should I say talking at each other? As I return to the table to relax and enjoy the end of this wonderfully crazy day, I see Dad going for the fruit salad. Yes, family is the source of our greatest joy, and maybe they do hear me—if only some of the time.

Nurses Whose Names Give Away a Tad Too Much
Andrew L.J. Heenan, RGN, RMN, BA (Hons)

- Eliza Katherine Gallagher works in Emergency. Her friends call her Kate, but when she initials a chart, she's "EKG".
- ... and Darcy Tuttle regularly signs charts with her initials—DDT

- The head of the nurse bank for Wells Hospital in Somerset was Sister Plaster—not bad for someone whose job was papering over the cracks in the service.
- Sister Pauline Iles works at Castle Hill Hospital—my source doesn't say if her friends call her "P"—or if she works in surgery.
- If your name was Diana, and you worked in Emergency ... would you let people call you "Di"?
- Isobel Risk, who teaches the HIV module in Scotland, signs off as I. Risk.
- An Accident and Emergency Department in Birmingham boasts a Nurse Payne
- Nurse Hacker scrubs regularly in a London Operating Department.
- Sister De'Ath walks the corridors of a hospice in Victoria.
- Does Annie Beaver still work in Obstetrics in New York?
- Mrs. Ake, a retired RN, was a specialist nurse in rheumatology.
- Kathy Foley was the head of the Catheter Insertion Team (back when they had those in the old days).
- Dr Hui (pronounced "Wee") was a urologist whose wife, a nurse, worked as his office manager. Her name was Pi (pronounced "Pee"). Nurse Cox worked for a different team.
- Chris Feely always favoured complementary therapies—especially therapeutic massage, while Nurse Fang was more at home with Cosmetic Surgery.
- Ed worked with a nurse, who was a nun, whose last name was Fuchs. He did not know how to pronounce her name—so he asked. And he wanted to die.
- Mary Slaughter could never get a post on the Surgical Unit, and Nurse Cutts was never the 'First Pick' Midwife.
- Sister Smallbones ran an orthopaedic ward in Stevenage.
- Sharon Ward—when she gets promoted—will be Sr. Ward.
- RN Melina works on the Endoscopy Unit (or did I make that up?) and Nurse Nurse—she goes where she's sent!

Reprinted with permission. Retrieved September 6, 2005 from www.realnurse.net. Edited from the original.

Beware: Mum Under Training

Philip Turner

I don't think that I was really listening when my mother confided in me. She intended to apply for nurse training. Either I was not listening or I simply did not realise the gravity of my situation.

Little did I know then that nursing training was synonymous with unpredictable mealtimes, very unpredictable maternal tempers, and even more unpredictable times at which the water pipes beneath the floorboards would clang as the good Samaritan plodded down the corridor to the bathroom, with a disruptive effect similar to that of a warning klaxon to those still in slumber. At the time of writing, Mum is serving a sentence in theatre so I get up before her, jumping spitefully on the water pipes to teach her.

At four in the morning of the first day of Mum's training, I was rushed to hospital for a minor operation and realised, with a start, that perhaps nursing was tougher than it looked. I was there for only a day and half but I learnt a lot. Sometimes the nurses seemed to have no individual personalities of their own, appearing to be a family of clones; at other times they seemed exactly the opposite. They certainly indulged in barbaric practices.

That was my first inside look at nursing life. It looked little better from the outside. Big books beeeeggggan to accumulate in the back room in which my mother studied. Her bedside stack of NTs grew until it had to be divided into two. Then three. Then four.

My grandmother came to stay more frequently, taking up the iron where Mum had left off, churning out socks, shirts, and turquoise uniforms at a phenomenal rate. She cooked, cleaned, dusted, hoovered, gardened, ironed, scoured, and slaved, and continued to work at her job in Leeds on top of this!

My father was forced to take to the kitchen, however, where he spent a good deal of time floundering around trying to prepare things that weren't fried, chilli, or shepherds pie. He became quite good at some things and is now learning to cook pasta dishes.

My brother and I remained little affected for the first few days, but then my mother's temper began to fray. After a month or two it was little more than a moth-eaten rag, and poor old Neil was dancing to the tune of a stinging wet dishcloth or a hail of soapy Brillo pads. I tried to keep out of the way but the occasional bit of shrapnel got me.

The first half hour after Mum returns is the worst. At first she spent it with her feet in the bath, but now she can spend it in the living room with them submerged in her foot spa, the irritating device that sends shockwaves up your legs from 20 feet away. Even this would not be so bad, but nursing seems to blunt the squeamishness of the students.

At meal times she will freely discuss diseases of the gastrointestinal tract while shovelling meatloaf into her own. No longer can I kneel or cross my legs in safety—no, it causes irreparable damage to the circulatory system. White bread, butter, chocolate, mints, cheese, and cream are all sure poisons, and pastry ranks with strychnine and arsenic. Her friends are little better. Friends of the family include an SRN and an RMN who insist that jogging shakes your brain loose, and that only by swimming 30 miles a week can one avert biological disaster.

The cats did not completely escape the ravages of nursing, either. They had to get used to going through periods of spasmodic growth when they would get fed twice as often as usual because everybody was getting up at different times, and harder times when they would be completely forgotten.

Mum was working on Christmas Day last year, and everybody else (as always) forgot to turn the video on at the correct times. The recipe for roast herby potatoes, a most jealously guarded formula, had to be passed on to another member of the family.

Of course, it is not all downhill. I now know where to go to find my adrenal gland, or who to ask if I have to do a project on the treatment of neoplasms. Things have settled into a routine once more, albeit after a shaky start. Sometimes having a nurse mother is a pain, sometimes it is a boon. Obviously, one must give and take on both sides. I once had to give her a fluorescent highlighting pen.

I must say that I have a very good reason for thanking her for taking up the job—without the extra money, I'd never have got my telescope. I am sure that more advantages will unveil themselves given time. It is certainly a job that I could never do; I can't even stand the smell in a butcher's. Still, it has been educational for us all, and I am certain that by the time my mum is ready to retire, she will be coming home to a family of gibbering hypochondriacs…

Woe to Be The Kid of Nurse!

Pat Veitenthal, RN, BSN

Woe to be the Kid of Nurse! Just ask my son. He's a rather verbal 10 year old who claims to be highly insulted that I never take his complaints of illness or injury seriously. Sound familiar? It infuriates him that each ache or pain is met with the gentle response, "Suck it up kid! I'm an ED nurse. I know what "hurt" REALLY looks like!" (Besides, aren't 10 year olds always either ill, injured, verbal, or highly insulted?)

These were, in fact, my very words to him when he fell off of his skateboard and landed on his left arm a while ago. Four days later, the EMT father of my son's playmate was kind enough to bring my son to me at work after noticing that he was not using his left arm at all. The EMT thought I would want to know this right away. He also thought that whatever happened was probably <u>his</u> kid's fault, and was interrogating him intensely. X-rays, of course, revealed that my son's left elbow was fractured in two places. Now I admit, I was perfectly willing to let the playmate take the rap, but my son, AKA The Informer, (who is a great deal like his father) arose piously from his seat, and announced within earshot of at least 3 neighboring states that his elbow had actually <u>been this way for 4 days,</u> and that his mother, <u>The ED Nurse</u> had known about it the whole time!

My colleagues then began asking my son if I had, in fact, PUSHED him off of his skateboard, Human Resources did a repeat background check, (and I swear I heard someone whisper Child Protective Services), and the heroic EMT stopped allowing his kid, who no longer speaks to me, to come over to our house. But since that silly little incident, I've noticed that my son has become very wise. He obviously began to study what I do for a living, because he has learned how to get attention. In fact, he's gotten so good at it that he has actually complained of chest pain (with shortness of breath yet!). Because he knows that it's triaged "Emergent"! Not when I was around mind you, but needless to say this terrified his father on more than one occasion, causing panicky phone calls to me at work…(but why should he believe my attempts at reassurance? After all, I missed the boy's elbow fracture…!) Not to mention what it did to his poor grandmother who still doesn't believe that I even graduated from high school, let alone two nursing schools! (Just because I played a little hooky in the 60's for Gosh sakes!) She's ready to mortgage her home to bribe Christian Bernard out of retirement for a Cardiac Consultation! Anyway, I gave my son a 6.425 for Originality, but told him he'd have to work on "cyanosis" before I was having any of it. But it does seem to be different for the Kids of Nurses, doesn't it? They do seem to have to "push the buttons" a bit harder than most kids. The RN who is the school nurse at my son's primary school is a friend of mine, and she tells me she can spot the Kid of a Nurse instantly.

She says they always know how to act really sick, rarely are really sick, and use phrases like "nucal rigidity"! Yeah, it can be rough to be a nurse's kid, but it sure isn't all bad. OK, so we miss an elbow or two every once in a while, but nurses' kids usually have "up to date" immunizations, and they're more likely to wear helmets, and seatbelts (and elbow pads which he had but didn't put on!) They're usually the first kids to learn their addresses and phone numbers, and they know that 911 is for emergencies long before they ever see it on TV! They know things like Stop, Drop, and Roll, and many of them know how to do CPR at a very early age. My son will even follow his 2 year old cousin around removing what he refers to as "Potential Airway Obstructions" from her path. Being the Kid of a Nurse is actually a pretty big deal when you stop and think about it. Just ask my 10 year old and he'll tell you. In fact, he'll tell you <u>anything</u> you want to know. Just <u>please</u> don't ask him about the change jar in his room labeled Future Therapy Fund...

Reprinted from Revolution: the Journal of Nurse Empowerment, ©1997; 7(1): 59 with permission of the author.

Shall I Tell You What I Think of You?

In the past, the physician/nurse relationship was clearly hierarchical, and physicians, as men, did not welcome women on their territory. Nursing was considered a custodiaww occupation, and nurses were considered the peers of patients economically, socially, and educationally. In recent years, nurses have enhanced their status through technical proficiency, though physicians still possess the clout in the medical profession. However, changes in this relationship are continuously evolving because of the increase in female physicians, the shortage of nurses, and the creation of new roles for nurses. So a time may yet come when both physicians and nurses will foster true collaboration and communication in the clinical setting.

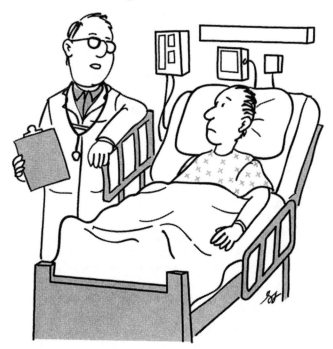

Of course your nurse loves you...
she's on Prozac–she loves everybody.

Praise Nurses and Your Patients Will Live Forever or Die Happy

Oscar London, MD

I've never met a nurse I didn't like. Well, once. But he didn't much care for me, either. Nurses come in all shapes, colors, and sexes and uniformly look terrific in white. And when they throw a dark-blue cape over their white shoulders, these angels take wing.

Working with a good nurse is one of the great joys of being a doctor. I cannot understand physicians who adopt an adversary relationship with nurses. They are depriving themselves of an education in hospital wisdom and are robbing their patients of round-the-clock loving care. A nurse who's miffed at a doctor can hardly be blamed for a certain coolness toward his patients—unless she's a saint, as not a few nurses are.

When I was a young doctor starting out in practice, I wasn't about to let a crusty RN tell this newborn MD how to practice medicine. Only after some years did I discover that a good nurse, like a good loaf of bread, is the staff of life, and the crustier the better.

Nurses have taught me to pull down the bedsheet over a patient so that the lower half of his body does not become a stamping ground for malpractice lawyers. (Decubitus ulcers, thrombophlebitis, perianal abscesses, and gangrenous toes are among the snappy tunes lawyers love to dance to.) A good coronary care nurse is one of the best cardiologists I'll ever meet. When she suggests stopping the quinidine, I stop the quinidine.

Nurses have taught me the intensive care that only compassion provides. Compassion is the conspiracy a good nurse forms with a patient to combat the inhumanity of hospitalization. ("When you get back from your barium enema, Mrs. Glick, I'll have your lunch and back rub waiting for you.")

I've had a nurse walk up to me and say the patient I admitted with "fever of unknown origin" had been bitten by a tick in Colorado the week before and was now probably in the early stage of Rocky Mountain spotted fever.... And what did the World's Best Doctor do after he wiped the egg off his face? He called up the nursing supervisor and praised the diagnostic acumen of that brilliant nurse to the skies. And when that nurse threw on a dark-blue cape over her white shoulders at 11 PM, she flashed me the most wickedly triumphant and grateful smile I've ever seen on the face of an angel about to soar up into the night sky.

Bugs are Not Funny Syndrome

Steven J. Schweon, RN, MPH
Ellen Novatnack, RN, BSN
Eileen O'Rourke, MT(ASCP), CIC
Susan Trout, RN, CIC

The recent identification of vancomycin-intermediate *Staphylococcus aureus* has reinvigorated legitimate fears in the infection control community that the microbe world is going amuck. This has had a dramatic impact on the behavior of a few of our fellow infection control professionals. Signs and symptoms include the following:

1. Contemplating a telephone condom for your office;
2. Taking a shower with a mask on to prevent legionnaire's disease;
3. Installing sinks at the front door so guests can wash before entering;
4. Washing your hands before and after going to the bathroom, just in case;
5. Demanding that waiters wash their hands before serving meals (and observing them do so);
6. Keeping a bottle of disinfectant spray handy to use on hand-held items between use;
7. Removing all blenders from your home;
8. Always carrying an extra pen in case someone asks to borrow one, so you can say, "keep it, I have an extra";
9. Requiring sedation when someone in an elevator sneezes without covering his or her mouth;
10. Always being prepared by carrying a "sinkless" handwashing agent wherever you go;
11. Placing handwashing stickers in your home bathroom as a reminder for family members and guests to wash up;
12. Waking up in a cold sweat from a nightmare involving mouth pipetting, eating, and drinking in the laboratory;
13. Development of rage attacks when making rounds and seeing a patient in Contact Precautions for methicillin-resistant coagulase-negative staphylococci.

3 Doctors & 3 Nurses

Three doctors and three nurses are traveling by train to a conference. At the station, the three doctors each buy tickets and watch as the three nurses buy only a single ticket. "How are three people going to travel on only one ticket?" asks the doctor.

"Watch and you'll see," answered a nurse. They all board the train. The doctors take their respective seats but all three nurses cram into a restroom and close the door behind them. Shortly after the train has departed, the conductor comes around collecting tickets. He knocks on the restroom door and says, "Ticket, please."

The door opens just a crack and a single arm emerges with a ticket in hand. The conductor takes it and moves on. The doctors saw this and agreed it was quite a clever idea. So after the conference, the doctors decide to copy the nurses on the return trip and save some money (being clever with money, and all that). When they get to the station, they buy a single ticket for the return trip. To their astonishment, the nurses don't buy a ticket at all. "How are you going to travel without a ticket?" says one perplexed doctor.

"Watch and you'll see," answered a nurse. When they board the train the three doctors cram into a restroom and the three nurses cram into another one nearby. The train departs. Shortly afterward, one of the nurses leaves his restroom and walks over to the restroom where the doctors are hiding. He knocks on the door and says, "Ticket, please."

Reprinted with permission. Retrieved December 6, 2004 from Medi-Smart, Inc. Website: www.medi-smart.com

Meeting Her Needs
Judy B. Smith, BSN

In 1994, our health department began serving as the primary care provider for thousands of patients who had previously only received public-health type services in our clinics. This switch to a "medical model" in our neighborhood clinics was quite a change not only for the patients but also for the staff who were more accustomed to providing chronic disease follow-up and preventive care, and now were being asked to provide acute care/primary care as well.

Because of this change, I was now a public health nurse in a primary care setting, working with the physician who was trying to meet the

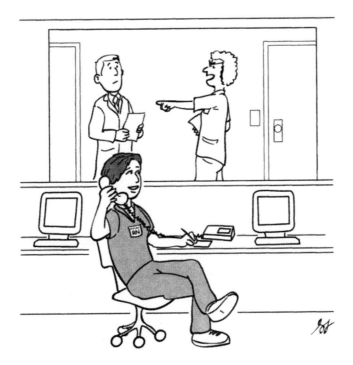

Do you want to speak to the doctor,
or the nurse who knows everything?

women's health needs as best he could. Not having done a lot of women's health previously, he was somewhat disorganized in his visit sequence but usually covered all aspects of care in a thorough, professional manner.

This particular day, the physician was completing a visit with a new, elderly patient. In his usual quiet way, as the patient was preparing to leave the examining room, he said offhandedly, "Oh, Ms. R., would you like to have a Pap smear today?"

Ms. R. appeared surprised and a bit confused because she was already dressed, had received her prescriptions, and thought her appointment was over.

"Why, yes, Doctor, that would be nice," the patient said.

I realized immediately that a communication error had just been made.

"Ms. R., the Doctor is asking if you want your PAP SMEAR done today—your test for cancer of the womb. You would need to get undressed again for that test," I tried to explain.

Ms. R. looked embarrassed and replied, "Oh, Doctor, I'm sorry. I thought you said PABST BEER! No, I don't want a PAP SMEAR today, thank you."

A New Speech Therapy Technique
Leslie Gibson, RN, BS

"I'm a speech therapist, and it was so embarrassing when I was work-ing on a head injury unit in South Florida. Unfortunately, a very hand-some young man about 25 years old had been admitted after a motor-cycle accident. He was experiencing urinary incontinence and while standing at the nurses' station, the staff were discussing the need to call the doctor for an order to insert a catheter. They really wanted to spare him the trauma, but none of their teaching efforts had been effective. One of the nurses recognized me and said, "Do you think you could help him use a urinal before we call the doctor?" Even though there was *no* order for speech therapy to see this patient, I agreed to stop into his room and attempt to help. Well, I showed him a urinal and pointed to where it needed to be placed. However, he just stared at me with a blank expression. (I thought to myself, I'm 52 years old. I've been happily married for 25 years, and raised two boys. Yes, I can do this!). So while reaching for the body part to be placed into the urinal... just at that moment... I had the feeling someone was watching me. When I looked up, his doctor was standing in the door-way. My heart was pounding, and I quickly removed my hand from his pants stating, "I'm the speech therapist!" The doctor responded by saying, "That's nice, but what are you trying to make talk?"

Skipping the Beat
Dorothea Kent

Entering a hospital room, a doctor was surprised to find his nurse holding the patient by both wrists. Thinking she was trying to take a pulse, he chided her for her unorthodox method.

"I'm not checking his pulse, Doctor," she replied through gritted teeth, "I'm checking his impulse."

Reprinted with permission from The Saturday Evening Post Magazine, ©March 1987, Saturday Evening Post Society.

A Doctor, a Nurse, and a Shredder

A nurse was leaving the hospital one evening when she found the doctor standing in front of a shredder with a piece of paper in his hand.

"Listen," said the doctor, "this is important and my assistant has left. Can you make this thing work?"

"Certainly," said the nurse, flattered that the doctor had asked her for help.

She turned the machine on, inserted the paper and pressed the start button.

"Excellent! Excellent!" said the doctor as his paper disappeared inside the machine.

"I need two copies of that."

Reprinted with permission. Retrieved October 21, 2005 from Medi-Smart Inc. Website: www.medi-smart.com

Fast! Warm! Fuzzy! Emergency!
David Wolman, PA-C

Stream of consciousness is what Freud viewed as a person's thoughts verbalized as uninhibitedly as possible. Here is the stream of my consciousness during a shift in the ED where I am employed. Freud needed a hundred volumes to explain this; I'll be brief. And forgive my honesty. It comes with the Stream.

Preparations Are Made
I am carrying two Chef Boyardee low-fat, low-cholesterol beef ravioli microwave meals, a product that recently received preliminary approval from the FDA as edible food. The packages are about the size of a hockey puck—truly lifesavers, with a 90-second microwave time. They enable me to spend only 15 minutes eating two meals during my 12-hour shift.

I have just logged in today's hours in the physicians' lounge. There are two books: one in which physicians record academic time, administrative time, on-call, CME, meetings, and vacation; the other is for PAs to record their work hours.

I have donned my white coat over blue scrubs and filled the pockets with essential clinical gizmos collected over the years. With accoutrements, the coat weighs 80 pounds, which keeps me from floating with joy at the thought of working windowless for 12 hours, not including a 45-minute commute, on the most beautiful day of the year.

No Sooner Do I Enter

A nurse approaches me. He has just graduated and he is very bubbly. He tells me that an 18-year-old male is in the waiting room. The patient had a 90% pulse ox on arrival but don't worry, the nurse reassures me, no wheezes now!

This patient has been here before, and ended up on a ventilator. His father, by the way, is an oncologist. Oh, the nurse concludes, and he takes asthmas medicine. The triage nurses have given the patient one nebulizer treatment out front. There are 20 patients ahead of him whose acuity ranges from plantar warts to blepharitis.

My brain, which hasn't yet been fed even a single helping of Chef Boyardee ambrosia, goes into high gear (picture a Hyundai with 200,000 miles): Low pulse ox. Asthma. No wheezes. Father is a doctor.... The longer I work in the ED, the more I think in simple terms. Because things can go down hill VERY SIMPLY.

My face drains of blood. I tell the nurse to put the patient in a room immediately. He asks me if it is OK to take the patient out of turn just because his father is a doctor. No, it is not okay to do this because his father is a doctor, I say. It is OK to do this because people who aren't breathing take preference.

The nurse is no longer smiling or bubbly. He retrieves the patient, puts him in Room 4, and informs me that he will be writing me up for, uh, something.

I don't greet the parents of the asthmatic boy—not because I am rude but because I can't help but notice that their son is using every accessory muscle I have ever seen and then some to breathe. His nostrils flare and he looks, well, a touch dusky. I inform my supervising physician that, without having examined the boy completely, my best judgment is that he is in imminent danger of respiratory failure despite a rejuvenating 2 hours in the waiting room.

Various orders are given. We start a nebulizer treatment but the nurse cannot find Atrovent to add to the albuterol because we are in the Fast Track area; emergency airway meds are in the core ED. We start an IV. We'd like to give steroids, but they are on back order from LL Bean. The nurse runs back and forth from the core, which is full, to our Fast Track, like someone in a nutty relay race on an old TV show.

Dad, the oncologist, is ominously silent but Mom, who reports that the boy was intubated previously in the ED, goes ballistic. Why would a mother be so emotional? I mean, her kid is going to need to be tubed any minute; they've been delayed for 2 hours; he is in the wrong part of the ED; and my supervising physician and I are missing only Curly to present a darn good imitation of the Three Stooges. Talk about overreaction!

We decide to move the patient to the core immediately. If they don't have room, that's their problem. (Actually, there are plenty of rooms—just not enough nurses to open them. We've played this game before.)

We'd like an oxygen bottle to move the patient. I run around looking for one. None in Fast Track. None in the core. The patient now does an excellent job of breathing with toe muscles. Finally, I find a bottle on a wheelchair out front. The patient in the chair has been waiting to have his emergent impacted cerumen cared for, so I shake off the thought that depriving him of oxygen will be brought up at the next QI meeting.

All we need now is an IV pole. None can be found. I grab the IV bag in my teeth, enhancing my professional demeanor, and away we go!

Now we're on a run with the stretcher at about 40 mph, the physician pushing and me steering. Mom swats me with her pocketbook to let off steam. The smacks are invigorating, a wonderfully refreshing beginning to my shift.

We arrive in the core. In seconds the patient is tubed. All is well. I'm grateful Dad is a doctor, because he knows how bad care can be. A normal person would have been shocked. (Mom? She called me later to apologize for the whacks and to thank me for quick action.) Only 15 minutes gone by, but I feel like I've lived through a millennium.

Can't Get Much Worse. Right?

That's my question as I sip lukewarm decaf tea. But then a colleague hands me an envelope. In it is a graph—one of those new graphs that people who go to school for medical administration learn how to construct. The note attached says that, according to the graph, which cannot lie, I'm not seeing the appropriate number of patients quickly enough.

Hey, 15 minutes for respiratory arrest! How fast do they want me to work? Oh I get it. They're talking about *real* Fast Track patients—suture removals, lacerations, abrasions, sprains, things you can really move quickly—meaning in 5 minutes. Problem is that half the time when I pick up a chart in Fast Track it's overflow from the core, meaning a very sick patient who fell through the triage sieve.

So this graph—created by someone who never sets foot in the ED for fear of stepping in something disgusting—this graph is irrelevant to what I do. This is the New World of Medicine. Things are measured and made more efficient and cost-effective. The only problem is that the things that are measured and made more efficient and cost-effective are not the things people do in an ED.

Another Chart, Another Medical Precedent

Migraine. Patient states she is allergic to just about every OTC and Rx analgesic approved for use in this country. Prophylactic meds don't work. Only Demerol works. Patient has listed an out-of-state physician.

I enter the room. The lights are out and the patient, in dark glasses, sprawls across the stretcher. No movement. I introduce myself quietly. She does not answer. Thankfully, however, she is accompanied by Tattoo-Man, self-made migraine expert, who will interpret her pain for her. Usually, he says, she gets 150 mg Demerol IM and 100 Percocets to go. I examine the migraineur and retire to my office.

I admit to a disagreement with Administration on this type of patient. Administration thinks that patient satisfaction is more important than the World Bank, that our job is to give the patient what she wants despite our medical judgment, give it to her fast, and be warm and fuzzy about it. My feeling is, yes, it is expedient to give the Demerol, but if the patient suffers from drug addiction, not headache, it is proper medicine to treat the real problem.

I call the patient's physician, dialing a number supplied by Tattoo-Man, but there's no listing for this doctor. Does this physician, in fact, exist? Maybe in Paraguay, but not the United States.

Uh-oh. My 15-minute turnaround time is about up. I feel like Lucille Ball trying to keep up with the conveyer belt of candy. (Nickelodeon reruns are my frame of reference.)

I explain that narcotics may only create rebound headaches—about as easily as explaining that a virus does not respond to antibiotics. Tattoo-Man fingers the Bowie knife on his belt; the patient under the sheet moans Chopin's Funeral March.

I confer with my supervising physician du jour (he's standing in for the regular Fast Track doc, who is at Disney World). He thinks Demerol is short and sweet. I must obey. Sure, I could raise a stink, but what would I get out of it? Be named designated complainer? We are a dependent profession. Nurses can refuse to perform orders contrary to their scope of practice; PAs cannot. We're physician extenders, not physician pretenders. There. I've said it and I feel better.

I order the Demerol. In the meantime, I schedule 20 PAs and the medical residents for moonlighting shifts over the next 3 months. I sketch out three articles for publication and give the PA student a quick summary of lupus. I long for my second Chef Boyardee, but it's too early. With gourmet food, you have to pace yourself.

All Along the Vertebrae

Next patient has had back pain for 10 years. I must cure it in 15 minutes. He tells me he had a herniated disc at L4-S1. Or is it L6-S12? He can't remember, but he's sure something is wrong with his L's and S's. I ask the obvious: Who is taking care of his back problems? Why is he *here* now? He tells me he is in pain, it's Saturday and his physician is not available, and he is allergic to everything except—hold on, don't tell me—Demerol! Should I consult my supervising physician? Or jump ahead to the obvious?

This time I get the patient's physician on the telephone. I am relieved to find that the doctor is real, and a very nice guy, too. He tells me that the patient has a substance abuse problem related to Vietnam (even though he never was there), his wife (the patient's wife), job stress (he in unemployed), and fibromyalgia, chronic fatigue syndrome, and temporomandibular joint dysfunction (all diagnosed by a chiropractor). He tells me to just give the Demerol and to ask the patient to see him on Monday.

I tell the nurse to hook up a large-gauge copper pipe to a huge vat of Demerol and start the IV.

Homeward Unbound

Eleven hours later, and I have taken care of fractured ankles, ingrown toenails, 12 children's fevers that would have responded nicely to Tylenol or Motrin had their parents given it, migraines, muscle aches, abrasions, burns, and a boxer's fracture in a guy who punched his refrigerator. I have stapled scalp lacerations, sutured another 10 or so, made splints for sprains and fractures (orthopods will only come in for patients who carry an extremity in a box), removed foreign bodies from eyes with a slit lamp and a needle, removed three foreign bodies from noses and two from other orifices, including a moth from an ear canal, called in dental consults on broken teeth and abscesses, treated toothaches with my Motrin-Tylenol with Codeine-Penicillin triad, x-rayed a penny in a baby's tummy, diagnosed external hemorrhoids and referred the patient to surgical clinic, diagnosed two cases of plantar fasciitis, given out 18 work excuses, written several thousand Motrin scrips (I exaggerate), and, yes, indulged in Chef Boyardee.

Buried in the mundane, I discovered meningitis, appendicitis, new-onset diabetes, cardiomyopathy in a 30-year-old whose only complaint was a cough that wouldn't quit, and active TB that presented as a cyst on the neck.

As I think about this on my way home, I notice flashing lights behind me. The state trooper recognizes me from the ED.

"Hey, *doc*, you don't have a license to speed."

I tell him he's absolutely right; I *don't* tell him that I am rushing home to catch a rerun of "ER." The work looks like so much fun there. Of course, if you add up commercial breaks and divide by the number of cases seen on an average episode—these people should be fired! Their graphs are terrible.

But the ratings are good. And that's what counts.

Help?
Michael M. Stewart, MD

When doctors doctor, and nurses nurse,

Most patients get better, though some get worse.

The system's not perfect, but one of the facts is

That no one is suing the nurse for malpractice:

She knows what her job is, and does it with grace,

While doctors make sure that she stays in her place.

Now nurses start doctoring: Junior Physicians?

Noctors? or Durses? Nurdocs? Nursicians?

What will their work be? And how shall we choose them?

How to be certain the public will use them?

And how to get doctors (traditional, staid)

To accept as their colleague this new Medi-Maid?

Problems aplenty, but what's even worse is:

If one of them's sued, they'll wish they were Nurses.

Creating the "Wow" Experience
Suzanne F. Ward RN, MN, MA, CNOR

I have worked in several ORs during my career. The ones I remember fondly are those where I had fun. Here are a few of my funny experiences.

Unfunny Boss
Our OR director was rather sober so when we heard she was making rounds to see how the new custom packs were working, the general surgery head nurse placed a sterile rubber spider on the side of the lap sheet. When the director walked into the room and asked how the new custom packs were working, the surgeon pointed to the spider and said, "Everything seems to be going well, but could you talk to them about the bugs we found." We all held our breath waiting to see her reaction. It only took a few moments for her to break into laughter.

Whining and Complaining Surgeon
Every time Dr. F operated, the whining and complaining were unbearable. We all dreaded working with him and didn't know how to tell him about this annoying characteristic. A new nurse suggested a fun and innocent prank. Just before Dr. F arrived in the OR, we taped empty 4 x 4 boxes over our ears. When Dr. F arrived, we didn't say word, just went about our work. When he noticed the boxes, he broke into laughter. After we all stopped laughing, we knew he got the message because the whining decreased.

Ordinary Surgeon Becomes Famous
One of our surgeons got involved with consulting for Hollywood movies. We thought he was becoming just a little full of himself. When we saw he was on the schedule, one of the nurses came decked out in false eyelashes, plastic lips, and makeup. As he entered the OR, she met him with autograph book in hand!

Reprinted with permission from Surgical Service Management, ©1999; 5(5): 6. Edited from the original.

Could We Start Again, Please?

In our fast-paced world we tend to communicate in all varieties of shorthand and acronyms. Acronyms should be easy to understand and remember but, unfortunately, that is not always the case. Some acronyms create endless confusion because they mean one thing to some people and quite another to others. The nursing profession is riddled with abbreviations and terminology that create extra barriers between them and their clients, and the door is wide open for the inadvertent misconception or even mayhem.

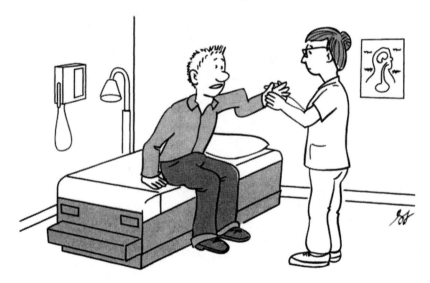

Is it broken or is it just fractured?

Help... I've Misplaced my Pronoun!

- The infant was handed to the pediatrician, who cried spontaneously.

- This 53-year-old white female was referred from a local medical doctor who has a long psychiatric history.

- The patient is a 90-year-old white female with multiple medical problems as well as severe osteoporosis that has been living with her daughter.

- The patient was the driver of an 18-wheel semi that was belted.

- He passed about a cup of bright red blood per rectum, which brought him to the emergency room.

- The patient ran into a deer on his motorcycle.

- I have suggested that he loosen his pants before standing and then, when he stands with the help of his wife, they should fall to the floor.

- The patient started taking Prozac given by her son who was a doctor one week ago.

- This 28-year-old woman comes to the emergency department shortly after a horse fell on her right leg while she was riding it.

- She was the driver of a vehicle which was wearing her seatbelt.

- Patient is a newborn infant delivered over an intact perineum which cried spontaneously.

- Patient's wife hit him over the head with an ironing board which now has six stitches in it.

- This 8-year-old came to the GU clinic with his mother who has had an absent right testicle since birth.

- This is an 83-year-old female who is unable to give her history due to dementia which is offered by her husband.

- She is using Demerol to relieve the pain which was given to her during her last hospitalization.

- This lady called saying her neck was increasing in size where we took it off.

- The findings were discussed with Dr. B and also the patient who joined us in the operating room.

- The patient resides in a nursing home which toppled over, resulting in a broken hip.

- The family history includes myocardial infarction in the father, who relates he died from this at an early age.

Heath, Diane S., ed [sic] Humor. Modesto, CA: American Association for Medical Transcription, ©1995. Reprinted with permission from the American Association for Medical Transcription.

Charting Bloopers: Spelling Errors
Patricia Iyer, MSN, RN, LNCC

- Admitting diagnosis: gang green.
- Patient with history of near drowning: patient had a sinking spell.
- Previously hospitalized at Mt. Cyanide (Mt. Sinai).
- Patient with urinary retention: "cant pea."
- Misses his mouth and drops foot all over his clothes.
- Had seeps of water.
- Had a deep pocket of puss lateral to rectum.
- Preoperative diagnosis: Stale Back Syndrome.
- This caused a gross of embarrassment.
- Patient needs a diaper for intoninence
- There was a perforation of a hallowed organ.
- Bold area on top of head.
- He went to see the chef of surgery.
- Heart rate of 140 beets per minute.
- Dressing changed ×1 for a large amount of serious drainage.
- Able to tolerate gentile range of motion.
- Patient able to giggle her toes bilaterally.
- Active woozing of wound.
- Pain and knumbness in neck/back/arms.
- Resident complained of an order coming from wound on buttock.
- Will wash face and upper torsos's daily.
- Fatal care given.
- Uptighted, could not sleep.
- Drowling from mouth.
- Ambulated with a steady gate.
- He had a fractured tibia plato.
- Uncomfortable with acks and pains.

- She was tossing and tuning.

- Patient remains wandered and agitated.

- The nurses have good rapoir with the family.

- She was probably identified and taken to the operating room.

- Patient is currently undergoing message therapy.

Reprinted with permission. Retrieved September 6, 2005 from www.medleague.com

Lost for Words

Jane Bates

The nurse's job? The nurse's task? No, that was not right. I was trying to find a synonym for 'role,' because in the piece I was writing I had used the word twice already. So I asked my husband. What did he come up with? 'Bap,' 'bun,' and 'teacake,' which goes to show that you can take the Yorkshireman out of Yorkshire, but never Yorkshire out of the man.

Finding the *mot juste* is also a constant challenge in the context of medicine. In fact, there ought to be a policy for linguistic health and safety. Take injections. Gone are the days when you could warn a patient by saying 'just a little prick' before you aimed a needle in their direction. But what expression can you use instead? No other word conveys the meaning as well. Jab, jag, and stab are too vicious—you wouldn't see the patient for dust. 'I am just going to inflict a little puncture wound' is far too verbose. 'Scratch' is not right and 'sharp scratch' just smacks of desperation because an injection does not feel like a scratch. But it does feel like a prick. Oh, all right, go on—laugh.

This precious use of language confused one of our receptionists last week, when a patient asked to be directed to the GUM department (GUM being the acronym for genito-urinary medicine). Owing to the misleading terminology, our colleague sent him to the orthodontic department, which is at the other end of the hospital.

It is not just language that counts; a typographical error can be a matter of life or death, which became apparent when a colleague had an outpatient appointment not long ago. It is the usual practice in our department to indicate that the patient is a hospital employee, but when we looked at the clinic list, we began to wonder if, for her, it was all too late. Because typed in brackets after her name was the word 'stiff.'

In the confusing world of eyes, where side by side lurk opticians, ophthalmologists, orthoptists and optometrists, there is a semantic accident waiting to happen. 'I went to see the op…, began a patient one day. 'The ophth…, the opt…,' he stuttered. It was not long before I started opthing and opting in sympathy. After a few minutes of what seemed like a joint attack of plosive hiccups, he said triumphantly: 'It was the optimist.'

At least he realised he had made a mistake, but not so the woman who said to me: 'I must tell you about my Appolypus.' Did she mean a medical condition, I wondered, or had she become romantically entangled with a bronzed Greek hero? Or was this some misbegotten horror created in a cauldron on a blasted heath somewhere—egg of cat, seed of parrot, that kind of thing? As I probed further, it became evident that she suffered from a nasal polyp. The word 'polyp' was not good enough for her, however. 'No,' she said, stubbornly, 'that is just a little one. Mine is bigger than that—it's an Appolypus.'

You can't argue with that kind of logic. You just have to reply with an understanding nursey kind of nod. But I was tempted to giggle when I overheard a woman on the bus the other day who was loudly proclaiming that she was about to have her kitten circumcised so she could let him out into the garden. I am sure she meant sterilised. Didn't she? In this case, whichever word you used, it would be all the same to the cat.

Reprinted with permission from Nursing Standard, ©2005; 19(27): 20-21.

The Study of "OLOGY"
Ruth Bay, CMT

1. ASTROLOGY	Small, colorful garden flower
2. CYTOLOGY	Vision
3. OSTEOLOGY	Sparkling wine
4. METEROLOGY	Shakespeare (iambic penta…)
5. ICHTHYOLOGY	Poison ivy rash
6. DERMATOLOGY	Der rug by der door to der haus
7. PATHOLOGY	Trails in the woods
8. BIOLOGY	Shopping
9. ZOOLOGY	Marlin Perkins
10. LITHOLOGY	The actress Taylor and her many marriages
11. ECOLOGY	Exclamations when you see a mouse

12. ORINTHOLOGY	Libido
13. ONCOLOGY	My aunt's husband
14. RADIOLOGY	CBS & NBC
15. PHYSIOLOGY	Carbonation
16. APOLOGY	Golden Delicious, Granny Smith
17. METHODOLOGY	A protestant denomination
18. OPHTHALMOLOGY	Dreadful things
19. CARDIOLOGY	Bridge and poker
20. HISTOLOGY	When you are "booed"

Heath, Diane S., ed [sic] Humor. Modesto, CA: American Association for Medical Transcription, ©1995. Reprinted with permission from the American Association for Medical Transcription.

Charting Chuckles
Jan Black, RN, OCN

At one time or another, every health care professional has probably charted a note or two that didn't come out quite right. These bloopers were collected from medical records across the country.

Cardiac
- Patient has chest pains if she lies on her left side for over a year.
- By the time she was admitted to the hospital, her rapid heart had stopped and she was feeling much better.

Musculoskeletal
- On the second day, the knee was better, and on the third day, it had completely disappeared.
- While in the emergency department, she was examined, X-rated, and sent home.

Neurologic
- Patient was alert and unresponsive.
- Healthy appearing, decrepit 69-year-old female, mentally alert, but forgetful.
- She is numb from her toes down.
- When she fainted, her eyes rolled around the room.

Gastrointestinal
- Rectal examination revealed a normal-sized thyroid.
- The patient had waffles for breakfast and anorexia for lunch.

- She stated that she had been constipated for most of her life until 1989, when she got a divorce.
- Bleeding started in the rectal area and continued all the way to Los Angeles.
- The patient was to have a bowel resection. However, he took a job as a stockbroker instead.
- Fleet enema given with stool hard as pine knots.
- Patient complains of indigestion since last night when he ate a stake.
- Patient passed flatus… two short, one long.
- Patient was seen in consultation by the physician, who felt we should sit tight on the abdomen, and I agreed.

Gynecologic/Urologic
- Examination of genitalia reveals that he is circus-sized.
- Indwelling urinary catheter draining clear yellow roses.
- Examination of genitalia was completely negative except for the right foot.
- Pelvic examination to be done later on the floor.
- Indwelling urinary catheter draining large amount of urine the color of American beer.
- MD at bedside attempting to urinate. Unsuccessful. (The physician was actually attempting to intubate.)

Social History
- The patient lives at home with his mother, father, and pet turtle, who is presently enrolled in day care three times a week.
- Patient was in his usual state of good health until his airplane ran out of gas and crashed.
- Examination reveals a well-developed male lying in bed with his family in no distress.

Miscellaneous
- The skin was moist and dry.
- Both breasts are equal and reactive to light and accommodation.
- The baby was delivered; the cord, clamped and cut and handed to the pediatrician, who breathed and cried immediately.
- Skin: somewhat pale, but present.
- I saw your patient today, who is still under our car for physical therapy
- Because she can't get pregnant with her husband, I thought you'd like to work her up.
- The test indicated abnormal lover function.

- If he squeezes the back of his neck for 4 or 5 years, it comes and goes.
- Discharge status: alive, but without permission.

Reprinted with permission from Nursing 97, ©1997; 27(12): 53.

More Charting Chuckles
Jan Black, RN, OCN

How's That Again?
- Occasional, constant, infrequent headaches.
- The patient left the hospital feeling much better, except for her original complaints.
- The patient is tearful and crying constantly. She also seems depressed.
- Patient has left his white blood cells at another hospital.
- She slipped on the ice and apparently her legs went in separate directions last December.
- Patient was released to outpatient department without dressing.
- Patient expired on the floor uneventfully.
- The left leg became numb at times and she walked it off.
- Patient lying on left side in no apparent distress with no complaints watching *Soul Train*.
- Diagnosis: uninhabited neurogenic bladder.

Patient/Physician Relationships
- The patient has been depressed ever since she began seeing me in 1983.
- I'll be happy to go into her gastrointestinal system; she seems ready and anxious.
- The patient will need disposition, and therefore, we will get Dr. Blank to dispose of him.
- Patient was admitted through the emergency department. I examined her on the floor.
- Between you and me, we ought to be able to get this lady pregnant.

History Lessons
- The patient has no past history of suicides.
- The patient's past medical history has been remarkably insignificant with only a 40-pound weight gain in the past 3 days.
- Coming from Detroit, this man has no children.

Just Follow the Directions

- I've suggested to the patient that he loosen his pants before standing and then, when he stands with the help of his wife, they should fall to the floor.

Patients Say the Darndest Things

- Patient states there is a burning pain in his penis, which goes to his feet.
- Patient refuses an autopsy.
- "Doc! Is it broke or just fractured?"

A Funny Thing Happened on the Way to the ED

Medical professionals aren't the only people who make the occasional misstatement. The following remarks were written on insurance forms by people involved in automobile accidents:

- The guy was all over the road. I had to swerve a number of times before I hit him.
- I pulled away from the side of the road, glanced at my mother-in-law, and headed for the embankment.
- An invisible car came out of nowhere, struck my vehicle, and vanished.
- In an attempt to hit a fly, I drove into a telephone pole.
- I was thrown from the car as it left the road. I was later found in a ditch by some stray cows.
- The indirect cause of this accident was a little guy in a small car with a big mouth.

Reprinted with permission from Nursing 98, ©1998; 28(5): 64. Edited from the original.

Medical Terminology 101

Darlene Sredl, RN, MA, MSN, PhD

Medical terminology is a pseudo-science that strives to break medical words apart in an attempt to examine what each syllable means independently. Then, the pre-translated syllables are put back together in an effort to make some sense of the whole word. Sometimes, however, even all the king's horses and all the king's men can't put the words back together again.

A complicating factor occurs in that many of the terms have a Latin or Greek origin—some also originate from other national languages. Here is an example of how the system works:

- Dosimitry—Dos/im/try—try to dose 'em

- Cilia—A girl's name
- Cyanosis—Poisoned by cyanide on an oasis
- Crossbite—To bite someone sitting across the table
- Fascia—A Nazi Communist
- Ganglion—Mascot from a group of troublemakers
- Corpuscle—An infection in the Marines
- Axis—A question as in "He always axis me what I want for my birthday"
- Ketone Bodies—Really fit people with high potassium levels
- Blastoma—A condition of accelerated flatulence
- Mast Cell—A jail on a boat
- Temporal Artery—Used until they construct a new art museum
- Sternotomy—A teacher who is really mad at me
- Pimple—French procurer
- Scratch test—Test for lice
- Seminal Fluid—Liquid used exclusively by Indians somewhere in the Southwest
- Reflex—Flexing a muscle repeatedly
- Café-au-Lait Spot—A great little coffee shop in Paris
- Friction Rub—A massage
- Free Radical—Out on Bond
- Heavy Metal—Rock band at the Café-au-Lait Spot
- Gnathic—A type of architecture
- Sub-Arachnoid—Under spiders
- Nanocephaly—Something Robin Williams said once
- Staph Albus—Caucasian work force
- Parotid—Administer parrots three times a day
- Phalanx—Back end of a horse
- Pariety—Two for tea
- C-Pap—"Yes, Dad" in Spanish

- Bi-Pap—"See you later, Dad" in English

- Prosoposternodidymus—I dunno, it's Greek to me, but now I'm obviously Russian to Finnish!

Top Ten Odd Medical Record Statements

10. The skin was moist and dry.
 9. The patient lives at home with his mother, father, and pet turtle, who is presently enrolled in day care three times a week.
 8. The patient was in his usual state of good health until his airplane ran out of gas and crashed.
 7. The patient was to have a bowel resection. However, he took a job as a stockbroker instead.
 6. I saw your patient today, who is still under our car for physical therapy.
 5. While in the emergency room, she was examined, X-rated and sent home.
 4. She stated that she had been constipated for most of her life until 1989 when she got a divorce.
 3. When she fainted, her eyes rolled around the room.
 2. She is numb from her toes down.
 1. The baby was delivered, the cord clamped and cut, and handed to the pediatrician, who breathed and cried immediately.

CPT Codes That Will Make You Chuckle
Leslie Gibson, RN, BS

- Perverted appetite—People who like to experiment with their food.

- Hysterical appetite—People who laugh at people who experiment with their food.

- Effort syndrome—For those who try and just can't get it right.

- Bad trip—For those vacations that didn't turn out the way you planned

- Best's disease—For people who think they're better than anyone else.

- Periodic breathing—As compared to not breathing?
- Buttonhole hand—For people who should use zippers.
- Holiday relief—What you are when the holidays are over.
- Excess gas—What happens when you overfill your gas tank.
- Hollow foot—Compared to a lead foot.
- Imperfect poise—Beauty contestant drop out.
- Infantile Hercules—A baby who can bench press his own weight.
- Seven-year itch—Wish to be single again after 7 years of marriage.
- Kink hair—Self-induced perm after jolt of electricity.
- Leprechaunism—For people who still believe there is gold at the end of the rainbow.
- Mirror writing—For those who fog up windows then write on them.
- Misplaced organ—Organ delivered in place of a piano.
- Negativism—For days when nothing goes right.
- Nodding of head—For 'yes' men.
- No diagnosis—When you don't know what is wrong.
- Overconscious personality—Politically correct term for brown noser.
- Overworked—Give this code to supervisor when you call in sick.
- Pancake heart—For those who dislike waffles.

Reprinted from Urologic Nursing, ©2004; 24(1): 62-63. With permission of the author. Edited from the original.

Premedicated Humor
Richard Lederer

An Austin, Texas, emergency medical technician answered a call at the home of an elderly woman whose sister had collapsed. As they were placing her into the ambulance, the lady wailed, "Oh lawdy, lawdy. I know what's the matter with her. She done got the same thing what killed her brother. It's a heretical disease."

The EMT asked what that would be, and the lady said, "The Smiling Mighty Jesus!"

When the EMT got the sister to the county hospital, she looked up the brother's medical records to find he had died of spinal meningitis.

A woman rushed into the lobby of a hospital and exclaimed, "Where's the fraternity ward?" The receptionist calmly replied, "You must mean the maternity ward." The woman went on, "But I have to see the upturn," Patiently, the receptionist answered, "You must mean the intern."

Exasperated, the woman continued, "Fraternity, maternity, upturn, intern—I don't care wherever or whoever. Even though I use an IOU, and my husband has had a bisectomy, I haven't demonstrated for two months and I think I may be fragrant!"

That same woman later became three centimeters diluted, and narrowly avoiding a mess carriage, she ultimately went into contraptions. Her baby was born with its biblical cord wrapped around its arm, and she asked if she could have the child circumscribed before leaving the hospital.

It is ironic that the humor in hospitals, emergency rooms, and doctors' offices—usually some of the scariest places—can be exceedingly hilarious. The giddy ghost of Mrs. Malaprop haunts medical halls and application forms, where we discover all manner of strange conditions, such as swollen asteroids (adenoids), an erection (anorexia) nervosa, shudders (shingles!), and migrating headaches…

A man went to his eye doctor, who told him he had a case of myopera and would have to wear contract lenses. That was a lot better than his friend, who had had a cadillac removed from his eye. Still, when he worked at his computer, he would have to watch out for harbor tunnel syndrome. He worried that his authoritis of the joints might be a signal of Old Timer's disease and fretted that a genital heart defect was causing a myocardial infraction and trouble with his duodemon.

Another man was in the hospital passing gull stones from his bladder while the doctor was treating a cracked dish in his spine. After the operation, his glands were completely prostrated. A hyannis hernia, hanging hammeroids, inflammation of the strocum, and a blockage of his large intesticle could have rendered him impudent.

We're not talking about just a deviant septum here. These symptoms were enough to give a body heart populations, high pretension, a peppery ulcer, and postmortem depression—even a cerebral hemorrhoid. But at least that's better than a case of headlights (head lice), sea roses of the liver…, or cereal palsy. Any of these could cause one to slip into a comma.

A woman experienced itching of the virginia during administration, which led to pulps all up her virginal area, and they had to void her reproductions. This was followed by a tubular litigation and, ultimately, mental pause. Mental pause can cause one to become a maniac depressive and act like a cyclopath.

She didn't worry about her very close veins, but she thought that a mammy-o-gram and Pabst smear might show if she had swollen nymph glands and fireballs of the eucharist. That's "fibroids of the uterus," and it's something you can't cure with simple acnepuncture, Heineken maneuver, or a bare minimum (barium) enema. Apparently, evasive surgery would be required. Afterward, she would recuperate in expensive care.

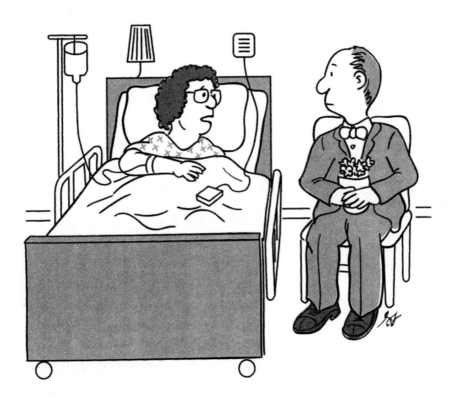

I am in here trying to pass gull stones from my bladder and now they tell me I have a cracked dish in my spine!

Quotable Quotes from Transcriptions
Marianne Janes, RNC, MHSc, NNP

Janet Pinelli, RNC, DNS, NNP

Verbal communication is easy to misinterpret. In hospitals, misinterpretation can be exacerbated by many factors. People with accents from around the world dictate radiology reports, operative procedures, physical examinations, discharge summaries, and other documents for transcription. Some mumble. Others speak very quickly. In addition, terminology varies greatly among disciplines and specialties. It is amazing that the transcriptionists on the other end of the phone are generally able to transform these cryptic messages into coherent printed form. The few errors that do occur, however, can make for humorous reading—although not for accurate descriptions.

The following fictitious discharge summary contains a compilation of transcription errors (in bold type) found on actual neonatal patient summaries over the years. Check your skills by correcting the errors. You'll find an answer key on page 86.

Dear Dr. Smith,

Thank you for accepting the ongoing care of Bobby Brown, who was discharged from the neonatal intensive care unit of St. Somewhere-else Hospital at 36 weeks corrected age.

Bobby was born to a 33-year-old $G_6A_3L_2$ mother at 24 weeks gestational age. There is a distant family history of **spidermolysis** bulosis, but no incidence in the immediate family. This mother's first infant had a clinical and chromosomal confirmation of karyotype 47 **excess** trisomy 21. Following that pregnancy, the mother experienced a **postmortem** depression. Her second child was a **dumb** neonate with spontaneous bilateral pneumothoraces requiring chest tubes and supplemental oxygen, but he has had no problems since the neonatal period. These children are now 12 and 10 years old. The mother subsequently had three spontaneous abortions in the second trimester, of unknown causes. She was understandably hesitant to become pregnant again, but decided on another pregnancy after reading several articles on the current status of perinatology and the improvement in infant **morality**.

This was an uneventful pregnancy, except for maternal **flue**-like symptoms three weeks prior to delivery. Two days prior to delivery, the mother had spontaneous **range of motion**. She was admitted to the labor and delivery ward for a high vaginal **tickle**. Fetal assessment was done, and the mother received betamethasone (Celestone) and antibiotics. Labor was **induced with forceps** due to a **crippling** breech presentation and a previous **V back** delivery. Delivery was by the vaginal root, and the **umbiblical** cord was **tied around the neck**. The infant was noted to be **sloppy** at birth and was resuscitated by head **banging** followed by **incubation**. His Apgars were 3 at one minute and 7.5 minutes.

The initial physical examination revealed an extremely premature infant who had **metric** growth restriction with head **spearing**. He was noted to have a **bulking** anterior fontanelle and a **flapping** forehead, which was felt to be due to *in utero* positioning. The remainder of his physical exam had **seizures** consistent with his gestational age. His **weight was 24 centimeters** and his **head circumference was 0.55 kilograms**.

The infant was admitted to the NICU and observed for the following problems:

1. **Respiratory.** The infant was intubated at birth and placed on a **semen** ventilator. His chest x-ray was compatible with **hollow** membrane disease, and he was treated with three doses of **exercise**. An **embolical** arterial line was placed to follow his **heart** gases. Bobby had severe respiratory **stress** but never developed a **phylothorax**. Chest x-ray at one week of age showed a moderate amount of **barrel trauma**. He received early dexamethasone for his chronic **lunch** disease. Bobby was extubated at the **age of 52** and required nasal pharyngeal CPAP until the **age of 71** due to his bronchopulmonary **dyspleasure**. He has been stable in room air for the past two weeks, with no apneas and no evidence of **dystacypnea**.

2. **Cardiac.** This infant had one echocardiogram, done at one week of age, that did not show a PDA but confirmed a **foramina valley**. There have been no other cardiac concerns.

3. **Sepsis.** On admission to the NICU, the infant had a sepsis workup and was **laced** on antibiotics. The blood culture demonstrated no **gross**, and antibiotics were discontinued in 48 hours. At two weeks of age, he had an infected IV site, which showed many **puss** cells and **grand** positive cocci. These results were phoned to the **nurd** immediately and antibiotics commenced. Culture confirmed a **staff** infection, which did not improve on cloxacillin, so the infant was switched to **Apresoline** for seven days. At six weeks of age, the infant had an elevated WBC, raising an initial concern for **cardiodialysis**, but blood cultures were negative. The infant has remained free from **inspections** since this time.

4. **Hematology.** Bobby was noted to have **thrombocytopenis** and **neutripnea** on his initial CBCs, most likely related to his growth restriction. These resolved without treatment. Bobby received **photoradar** for three days in the first week of life for physiologic jaundice. He has received two blood transfusions for anemia.

5. **Hernias.** The infant developed **bilingual** hernias, which were surgically repaired under **coddle** anesthesia three weeks ago.

The patient was **raped** and prepped for this procedure in the usual manner. Because his parents had wanted Bobby to be circumcised, his **urethra** was removed during the same surgery. Recovery was uneventful.

6. **GI/Fluid Balance.** The infant was initially hypoglycemic **and fed with sticks.** He responded to total **parental** nutrition by **deep tendon fusion.** The umbilical **vessels** were removed on day 7 of life, and a PICC was inserted into the right **lung** saphenous vein. This was removed when he was tolerating full oral feedings. Early in his stay, the infant had a low serum sodium, which was felt to be **delusional.** His electrolyte status had been otherwise normal. Bobby had one abdominal ultrasound done on day 3 of life in response to oliguria. The ultrasound showed that the **rental** structures were normal. The oliguria subsequently resolved without treatment. Because of some concern about **perianal** asphyxia/low one-minute Apgar, the infant was not fed until he had passed several **bowl** movements. The infant was fed with **express** breast milk by gavage, which he tolerated without problem, until he was able to establish **beast** feedings. For the past two weeks, Bobby has been **winking** and demanding feedings every 3-4 hours. He is presently gaining **3,250** grams per day. He demonstrated **catchup** growth, and his weight on discharge is 2,785 grams.

7. **Neurologic.** Bobby had several **three-wall** ultrasounds while in the NICU. The initial ultrasound on the second day of life showed a **terminal** matrix hemorrhage. Follow-up ultrasounds showed **normal** areas of hemorrhage with no **hydrosyphilis.**

8. **Retinopathy of Prematurity.** The infant has been seen three times by our ophthalmologist for **risen up the prematurity.** His eye exams showed **normal ocular pathology.** Because his retinas are not yet fully vascularized, he has a follow-up appointment in two weeks to monitor his retinopathy **or** prematurity.

9. **Discharge.** Bobby Brown was discharged home today 36 weeks corrected age, **with his parents in a car seat.** He is on *ad lib* demand **beast** feedings, with **Polyvision** and vitamin D supplements. His pediatric care will be provided by Dr. W. Smith. His only **timing** problem is his retinopathy **is** prematurity.

Good luck with this child's **car.**

Dictated by: TL Jones, RNC, NNP

Answers for *Quotable Quotes from Transcriptions*

Spidermolysis = epidermolysis
Excess = XX
Postmortem = postpartum
Dumb = term
Morality = mortality

Flue-like = flu-like
Range of motion = rupture of membranes
Tickle = trickle
Induced with forceps = induced and the infant delivered with forceps assistance
Crippling = footling
V back = VBAC (vaginal birth after cesarean)
Root = route
Umbiblical = umbilical
Tied around the neck = tight around the neck
Sloppy = floppy
Head banging = hand bagging
Incubation = intubation
7.5 = 7 at five
Metric = symmetric
Spearing = sparing
Bulking = bulging
Flapping = sloping
Seizures = features
24 centimeters = 0.55 kilograms
0.55 kilograms = 24 centimeters
Semen = Siemen's
Hollow = hyaline
Exercise = Exosurf
Embolical = umbilical
Heart = art. (arterial)
Stress = distress
Phylothorax = pneumothorax
Barrel trauma = barotrauma
Lunch = lung
Age of 52 = on day 52
Age of 71 = day 71
Dyspleasure = dysplasia
Dystacypnea = dyspnea
Foramina valley = patent foramen ovale
Laced = placed
Gross = growth
Puss = pus
Grand = Gram
Nurd = nurse
Staff = staph
Apresoline = vancomycin
Cardiodialysis = candidiasis
Inspections = infections
Throbocytopenis = thrombocytopenia

Neutripnea = neutropenia
Photoradar = phototherapy
Bilingual = bilateral
Coddle = caudal
Raped = draped
Urethra = foreskin
And fed with sticks = as noted on Dextrostix
Parental = parenteral
Deep tendon fusion = intravenous infusion
Vessels = catheters
Lung = leg
Delusional = dilutional
Rental = renal
Perianal = perinatal
Bowl = bowel
Express = expressed
Beast = breast
Winking = waking
3,250 = 3 to 5 (three to five)
Catchup = catch-up
Three-wall = cerebral
Terminal = germinal
Normal = no more
Hydrosyphilis = hydrocephalus
Risen up the prematurity = retinopathy of prematurity
Normal ocular pathology = no ocular physiology
Or = of
With his parents in a car seat = in a car seat, with his parents
Beast = breast
Polyvision = Poly-vi-Sol
Timing = remaining
Is = of
Car =care

Reprinted with permission from Neonatal Network, ©1999; 18(4): 59-60, 74.

My Trips Over the Language Barrier
Debora A. Wilson, RN, MN

Communicating across language and cultural barriers is a challenge
that's always appealed to me. And I assure you, I've made progress
since the first time I attempted it...

A physician had asked me to translate his words into Spanish for a patient who was having abdominal pain. Unfortunately for all of us, they don't teach you how to translate "adhesions," "lactose intolerance," and "gallstones" in your run-of-the-mill Spanish class. I'm certain that were I a patient in a country where English is not spoken routinely and a nurse calmly explained that I had a rock by my liver, the concept of gallstones would not occur to me right off. Gratefully, however, the patient nodded to me and smiled.

I was reminded of a story my cousin tells about a physician who had little command of English who tried to tell her that she had a dermoid ovarian cyst (you know, the type that sometimes grows teeth or hair). Said the doctor, "It's like a little person." My cousin imagined a little man with glasses and a briefcase standing on her ovary trying to figure out what he was doing there.

Looking back over other transcultural *faux pas* that crossed my lips, I realized that most fall into one of the following classifications.

When words sound like what you mean—but aren't. I'm sure I'm not the only student of Spanish who's said she was *embarazada* for "embarrassed," only to find out she'd been telling people that she was pregnant.

When phrases don't transliterate. As a nurse who tries to be sensitive to the psychosocial aspects of my patients' health, I'd often ask them how things were at home. After many blank looks and no useful responses, I realized that I was asking them, literally, how *things* were at home, as in "How is the sofa?" or "How is your dishwasher?"

Once I was talking with a pregnant patient about her excellent memory. Without thinking, I muttered, "You are like an elephant." Her horrified response made me realize that not only does no pregnant woman want to be compared with a multi-tonned animal, but that the English idiom makes no sense in Spanish.

Another idiom that has no Spanish counterpart is "I changed my mind." A few odd looks from my patients prompted me to ask my Spanish instructor what I'd been saying wrong. Apparently, I'd been implying that I'd had a brain transplant.

When an innocent-sounding word turns out to be suggestive. I'd spent months innocently directing patients to a receptionist to make another appointment—until a staff member overheard me. Apparently, I'd been inadvertently instructing them to engage in crude behavior.

Sometimes, such mistakes can prompt constructive change. In my one and only attempt to teach a class on contraception to couples, I used quite a few Spanish words that are not to be mentioned in mixed company. Suddenly and magically, the funds for hiring a bilingual health educator appeared.

When patients speak slang—and you don't. A patient with abdominal pain told me that the pain subsided when she got upset and "threw pens." Rather than asking her how many pens she had to throw to control the pain, I called in our bilingual administrator. My patient had been talking about passing gas.

As a nurse practitioner, I enjoy working with my patients and learning about their culture. In three years, I've refined a lot of my Spanish, but every time I'm ready to congratulate myself, someone comes along to humble me. Last week, for example, a patient I hadn't seen for a year told me my Spanish had improved quite a bit. Just as I started to feel complimented, she added, "Last year, you couldn't speak it at all!"

Reprinted with permission from American Journal of Nursing, ©1989; 89(12): 1718.

Clarification, Please!

- Chest x-ray shows sinus rhythm.
- EKG of the ankle showed a small ossicle.
- Electrocardiogram showed fibrosis in the right lung.
- Examination of the abdomen revealed mitral regurgitation.
- The ears are normal and move well.
- Call the doctor back if you still have problems after the swelling between your nose decreases.
- EKG showed normal sigmoidoscopic exam.
- Speculum was inserted between the eyes.
- Barium enema showed obstruction of the mid-esophagus.
- IVP reveals slow heart rate.
- Patient was placed on a low-salt, high-food diet.
- She was treated with Mycostatin oral suppositories.
- Her arm was in a long-leg cast.
- The patient had a low-grade temperature of 108.
- Her nose and pharynx are with full range of motion without any adenopathy.
- I recommended that she be placed on heparin beginning in 12-18 hours and after a repeat CT scan is done to rule out the possibility of any blood being present in the head.
- Patient: 45-year-old white male
  - Specimen: Hernia sac
  - Diagnosis: Products of conception
- Patient received in one container, labeled *hernia*.
- … with the patient awake and alert under general anesthesia.
- This 7-month 3-day-old baby weighed 117 pounds.

- The patient was started on life-threatening treatment.
- Patient had carcinoma of the prostate and a penile transplant.
- *Patient with tonsillitis:* If he develops any difficulty swallowing or sign of asymmetry, he will follow up like an abscess.
- CHIEF COMPLAINT: Headaches for 4 years.
  PRESENT ILLNESS: The patient has had left-sided headaches for more than 12 years, starting approximately 3 years ago. She required considerable analgesic abuse. She is admitted for definitive surgical treatment; the plan is for excision craniotomy.
- … grew *Klebsiella pneumoniae*, which was resistant to cefoperazone. Therefore, tobramycin was discontinued, but patient was maintained on one antibiotic, namely cefoperazone.
- He states he has some disks in his neck, but this cannot be substantiated.
- Her postoperative course was fairly unremarkable, although she was noted to have no return of her heart rhythm.
- The patient's urine intake was adequate.
- Bleeding was again achieved with electrocautery.

Heath, Diane S., ed [*sic*] Humor. Modesto, CA: American Association for Medical Transcription, ©1995. Reprinted with permission from the American Association for Medical Transcription.

Document — Don't Duckamint!

Pat Veitenthal, RN, BSN

Up until now, I admit I've been secretly amused by the way patients so easily mispronounce medical terms—no matter how often they've heard them said correctly. I've often grinned or grimaced at "high hernia," bronical" infections, pain in the "groinal," and, one of my favorites, heart "palipations."

I've heard complaints of "vomiking" all night from the "intesticle" flu, and requests for "teknis" shots. Recently, one of my patients told me she was taking "Premium" for menopause, and another said she was taking "Zanattack" for ulcers. As you might expect, she arrived by ambulance with the "sireen going."

I can live with this, but when nurses mispronounce, misspell, or misuse words or phrases—particularly when it comes to documentation—I WORRY! We are, after all, supposed to be reasonably well educated and should know better. Today, when nursing positions are threatened by the use of unlicensed personnel and managed care, it is certainly NOT the time for nurses to appear ignorant!

Patients can be reeducated, or least forgiven, but there is no excuse for nurses when they misuse terms or document data according to less-than-perfect standards. Over the years, I've collected some particularly deplorable examples of the misuse of terms. Hopefully, they will serve as a reminder of the importance of professional documentation.

From Triage:
- "Here for suture removal. Three sutures. Back of head intact." (Thank Heaven!)
- "C/O low back pain. Hx of ruptured dick." (Uh… and this was the *correction* from 'disk'!)
- "Pain in Rear." (I wasn't sure if this was a patient complaint, or a personality assessment. It turned out to be a right *ear* infection!)
- "Pt. requesting Demerol. Looks like he needs it."
- "S/P tooth extraction. Now c/o air pocket symptoms." (The term is dry socket!)
- Subjective: "Bitten by a snake. No movement, 17 in., multicolored, flat head." (My friends, here you have a classic—the nurse assessed the SNAKE!)

From Nurses' Notes:
- "LMP: Constantly, since age of 13." (Pt. was 42. Whew.)
- "Pt. left without being seen. Will return later with leg if not busy." (I don't even know where to begin with this one.)
- "Currently minastrating with period."
- "Pupils equal and photosizing to light."
- "Pt. states she is vomiting. Will observe for truth." (How Zen!)
- "Two valium missing from stock. Supervisor notified that I didn't do it."
- "Scrotal support applied as ordered. He was a perfect fit for me."

Reprinted from Revolution: the Journal of Nurse Empowerment, ©1996; 6(3): 44 with permission of the author.

Acronyms Anon

Nurses are in hot water over their note-taking. The angels, it seems, have a rather dark sense of humour and use a variety of less than flattering acronyms to describe their patients' conditions. BUNDY stands for But Unfortunately Not Dead Yet. FLK means Funny Looking Kid, PIN is a Pain In the Neck. If they are found out they will face disciplinary action, according to the UKCC (The United Kingdom Clerical

Controllers, aka the UK Central Council for Nursing, Midwifery and Health Visiting).

Nurses are, of course, just following the lead given by doctors. FLK is a classic piece of GP note-ese, along with SIG (Stroppy Ignorant Git). The BMA (Beware Malevolent Acronyms) has on several occasions warned doctors not to add such personal annotations to their patients' medical records but without much success. GPs probably reason that, since no one can read their handwriting anyway, they are safe from legal redress.

Soldiers also use acronyms as part of their defence. SNAFU—Situation Normal, All Fouled Up, or something along those lines—was a universally accepted description in the second world war. SAPFU—Surpassing All Previous Foul-Ups—marked a deterioration in affairs.

The black humour of the medical, as much as the military, world is a fact of life; or more properly a way of coping with death. Nurses mock the emotional involvement of the staff in the TV series Casualty: when death and disaster are your daily currency, you can't afford to grieve. They are not superhuman and the in-jokes and barbed references seem to act as an outlet, almost a catharsis, a way of laughing in the face of routine suffering. Angels are helpful after death; sane, rational, focused professionals are more useful pre-BUNDY.

Mr. Jones' Diary

Mr. Jones: I heard that Mr. Wallace had to stop operating in the middle of a case because his foreign scrub nurse couldn't understand English.

Sister: Her English is impeccable. She just doesn't speak 'surgeon' yet.

Mr. Jones: Are you suggesting that we surgeons speak a language of our own, just like some primitive tribe?

Sister: That's exactly what I'm saying.

Mr. Jones: Nonsense. I've never heard anything so ridiculous.

Sister: Well, there are some general phrases that all surgeons use, like *'Sister, how many nurses have you got on the late shift?'* which means *'Sister, I'm thinking about splitting my list and opening up a second theatre;'* and *'I've got to go to a meeting'* means, *'I'm off to do a bit of private work but I'll be back before the end of the list.'* And then, of course, there are different dialects.

Mr. Jones: Different dialects?

Sister: Oh, yes. Surgeons in different specialties speak different dialects. I can understand 'orthopaedics,' 'general' and 'plastics' but I'm afraid that my 'obstetrics' is a bit rusty.

Mr. Jones: So now you're trying to say that we mean different things, depending on our specialties?

Sister: Yep, for example, in 'plastics', *'Can I have a 6-0 nylon?'* means, *'I will sit here quite happily irrigating this wound while you search this theatre, the one next door and finally the store cupboard for a 6-0 nylon.'* Conversely, in 'vascular', *Can I have a 6-0 nylon?'* means, *'I want a 6-0 nylon right now and if I don't get it right now I will scream and shout until the theatre manager has to come in and calm me down.'*

Mr. Jones: I see what you mean. I apologize, Sister. I think you're right.

Sister: Now, you've got me on that one, Mr. Jones. I don't think I've heard that particular phrase before.

Reprinted with permission from British Journal of Perioperative Nursing, ©2003; 13(2): 55.

Night and Day 6

Smiling your way through work is a preposterous idea, though it can work wonders from time to time. Our rose-colored glasses should not be in a drawer gathering dust. It may be true that most days we are so concerned with survival that we no longer have the luxury of seeking contentment and bliss, but we owe it to ourselves to reach for the stars. It may mean chasing our dreams, whatever they may be, with all our heart and soul, and keeping the chase until we reach them. The key to success in our chase is learning to embrace the unknown, work the mistakes, and tolerate the pain.

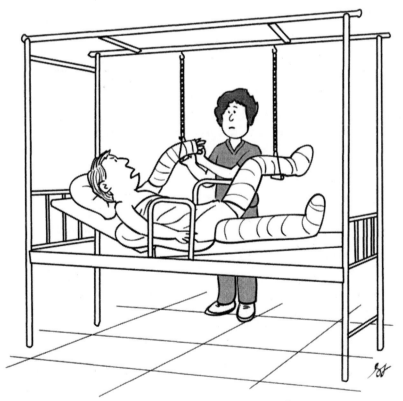

At the rates I'm paying, what do you mean when you say
you don't have a wine list?

Finding Humor in Our Workplace
Sharon P Hall, RNC

In my 30 years as a perinatal nurse, I've collected or heard some terrifically funny tales about us, our patients, and the services that we perform. And sharing them with others is especially fun. Here goes:

Par for the Course
A childbirth educator relays the story of a room full of pregnant women and their partners for a Lamaze class. The instructor was teaching the women how to breathe properly, along with informing all of the partners how to give the necessary assurances at this stage of the plan.

The educator then announced, "ladies, exercise is good for you. Walking is especially beneficial. And gentlemen, it wouldn't hurt you to take the time to go walking with your partner!" The room got really quiet. Finally, a man in the middle of the group raised his hand and asked, "Is it all right if she carries a golf bag while we walk?" Yeah, right!

The Right Word, Please
As perinatal nurses, we are often amused when patients tell us they would like "their epidermal" (epidural) or that they "are here this morning to be seduced!" (induced). I will always remember the look on one mother's face when my colleague told her "the baby will be placed under the hood."

It's also been related to me that there were two 10-year-old boys who were overheard discussing birth at the entrance to the LDRP suite, and one said, "They call it a delivery room, but it's really a take-out place." One pediatric nurse overheard a little girl tell her brother in the waiting room, "He gave me a shot for the mumps, measles, and rebellion." And last, there was that time when I went to give a fetal monitoring lecture at a local hotel and the marquee read "fatal monitoring."

Charting Chuckles
The strangest things get written down in our effort to tell the whole story of the women for whom we provide care. Describing a woman recovering from an epidural, one nurse wrote, "the left leg remains numb at times, but she walked it off." Or "at the time of pregnancy, the woman was undergoing bronchoscopy." I once read, "she was treated with Mycostatin or suppositories." Or how about, "both the patient and myself report the passing of flatus."

One nurse wrote, "the patient has contractions if she lies on her right side for several months." One admission was noted as "healthy-appearing, decrepit 69-year-old female, mentally alert but forgetful."

And finally, "The pelvic examination was done on the floor." I once wrote, "the patient was admitted to the hospital on the day of admission." I left it just to see if anyone would notice—and of course, no one did!

I've also seen some good stuff written by our medical colleagues: "We have been sitting on this patient for some time." How about, "this unfortunate 60-year-old woman has been seen by me for 10 years." Also, "patient was dismissed home without dressing;" "Mrs. Jones was admitted with diarrhea from the ER;" and "the patient has never been pregnant and denies any reason for this."

Women Say the Funniest Things

One nurse related that she gave a woman a referral slip for the GI clinic. The woman stated, "This must be wrong, I was never in the military service." A nurse fielding a phone call from an anxious lady was asked, "How long does it take to get over gamma globulin?"

One woman, waking up from general anesthesia in the recovery room, was told by the nurse, "You have a beautiful baby boy!" The mother said, "I do? Well what is his name?" This one from a frail, elderly lady on admission: "I've been in this hospital so often, it's like home. I know everyone. What's your name?"

Overheard in the surgical suite: "Why can't I wear lipstick to surgery? I'm having my uterus removed, not my lips!" One primiparous woman after unloading two suitcases, a video camera, two still cameras, a 'goody bag,' and a potpourri pot, smiled and joyfully stated, "My contractions are 15 minutes apart, I think I'm in labor."

An elderly lady, being questioned by a nurse regarding her activity, reported "lately, I've gotten into transcendental vegetation."

A patient once told me that she had been having repeated bouts of Braxton-Hicks contractions in her 39th week of pregnancy. One night, as she tossed and turned in discomfort, her husband turned over and, placing his mouth very close to her abdomen, stated, "Stay in your womb and don't come out until we tell you."

You Know It's Been a Bad Day When...

- The nurse manager says, "we have a few changes..."

- No one shows for mother-baby class

- Your patient passes out in the bathroom after a Fleets enema, and you gently slide her down your legs where she sits on your shoes

- You drop your pager in the toilet.

Reprinted with permission from AWHONN Lifelines, ©1998; 2(6): 64, 63. Edited from the original.

Nursing Realities
Diane Sears, RN, MS, ONC

A patient was admitted in a poor state of hygiene. The nurse tech stated, "There is so much dirt between his toes, I could grow potatoes."

You consider it a foreboding omen that, while sleepily applying your makeup in a hurry to get to work, you sneeze and your mascara wasn't dry yet.

You plan various tactics of human annihilation, when you come back to your desk and find someone else in your chair.

The new specialist can't understand why you have reported him to your supervisor because he has changed your patient's orders 5 times in one hour, reversing himself three times.

You fantasize being Samantha, the Bewitched Nurse, twinkling your nose and curing all in your care.

The nurse was having such a bad day, she prayed for her own death.

Wishee washie versus swish and swallow.

A RN had just received a cookie bouquet from a grateful patient with her name on it. She's in the process of admiring it with her co-workers, when the grandson of a retired employee, cruises by and the retiree watches as he takes a bite out of one, doesn't like it, and throws it away, ruining the bouquet.

Patient calls to "have this jack removed from my leg." It was a continuous passive motion machine.

Nurse receiving report complains to the nursing supervisor that "a nurse had called her patient a twerp." The reporting nurse had explained the patient "had a TURP."

The nurse thought the MD wanted her to RSVP him instead of the diagnosis, RSV.

Founded in 1983, there are Workaholic Anonymous Chapters, all over the United States.

Reprinted with permission from Oklahoma Nurse, ©2005; 50(1): 23.

Desperate Strategies for Last-Minute Staffing
Sybil Kaufman, RN, CS, MS

It's 2 PM on Friday and you're determined to finally leave work on time. If you get home late again:

- Your spouse will file for divorce
- Your kids might not recognize you
- Your good friends will desert you.

You foolishly think, "Aha, I'm going to do it. I'll be outta here soon—no sick calls!" Then your pager goes off, and you recognize the number as an outside call. You say to yourself, "I'm done. Who will I ever find to work tonight? I should've been a vet tech."

If this scenario is all too familiar, help is on the way. But first you must put aside all traces of self-respect, pride, and conscience. Prior experience in procurement is useful, although experience in selling used cars will do.

When there's nothing left of your superego, you need to remind yourself that you're not Florence Nightingale. Compose yourself. Focus on your goal—to find a nurse for the evening.

You Realize She's Ill, But...

Return the call on your pager. Yes, it's Ms. Smith, who hasn't called in sick in 3 years. She tells you in a hoarse, ill tone that she's just been diagnosed with strep throat, has a 102° F fever, and is so sorry but... Don't let her finish the sentence. Say, feigning sympathy and sincerity, "Now Ms. Smith, I know you feel ill so I'll:
- Let you come in 1 hour late
- Give you all the light patients and no admissions
- Have a car service pick you up and take you home."

If Ms. Smith demurs with a comment such as, "But I'm contagious," you must reply, "Remember those TB mask fittings?" If she drops the phone and her husband picks it up to say his wife appears to be having febrile seizures, mutter a hasty, "So sorry, but also tell her I'll approve her time-off requests for the next year," and continue making promises. You never can tell—she might just call you back.

The Per Diem Haggle

If that doesn't work, your next likely candidates are, of course, your day staff. Throw caution and your budget variance to the wind. Try to forget that they're exhausted and looking forward to spending the evening with their friends and families. Don't do the math and calculate that some of them will earn $125 an hour. For this reason, approach the most senior nurse first.

Go through your previous list of promises. If that doesn't work, try saying, "If you work this evening, I'll:
- Approve as professionally relevant your request for time off the week of December 25 to attend the conference 'Psychosocial Aspects of the Baxter Pump' in Hawaii
- Give you comp time off on Sunday, allow you to use your emergency free days for the next two Saturdays, and send your union rep a bouquet of roses."

- Still no takers? Then give it your best shots, "If you work this evening, I'll also:
- Permit you to resign from the Policy and Procedures Committee
- Permit you to resign from the QA Committee."

Still holding out? Then it's time to review your list of per diems. (I realize you probably don't have a list. But maybe you keep a folder of paper scraps scribbled with barely legible names and numbers, the result of past desperate calls to colleagues begging for the names of their per diems.)

Remembering that time is money, but not *your* money, go immediately to the nurse on your list who's almost always available. You know, the one your staff nurses have told you they'll never, ever work with again. The one who, if you hire her, almost certainly will force your staff to file three protests of assignment?

Make the call. Hire the nurse.

Once You Reach Your Car...

Then, when your staff is in report muttering about working short for the umpteenth time, put on your coat. Breeze into the report room and casually, say, "I found someone to work." And slip out the door before they can ask "Who?" Enjoy your evening.

This flight strategy also applies to posting schedules, which you should only do Friday afternoons as you're leaving. Better yet, hand them to the unit clerk with instructions to give you at least 10 minutes lead time to get to your car before posting them.

Although these measures may make sanity and the nurse manager seem paradoxical, you can reflect on this puzzle from the comforts of home.

Reprinted with permission from Nursing Management, ©2000; 31(1): 35.

Top Ten Reasons (and more) Why I Want Star Trek's© Medical Beds in My Unit!

Tom Trimble, RN, CEN

10. The patient never has to be helped into or out of bed, nor even undressed.
9. The patient doesn't have or need any I.V. lines, tubes, or monitor cables.
8. The patient doesn't need a footstool, to be pulled up in bed, or even have a siderail.

7. The patient never needs to be fed, and never needs to be bathed.
6. The patient never has an excessive number of visitors.
5. The patient never vomits, urinates, defecates, or expectorates.
4. The patient <u>will</u> get up cured at the end of 46 minutes, unless killed off in the first five minutes of the show to entice you into watching the remainder of the program. He will not need a wheelchair for discharge.
3. The patient rarely needs translator services arranged.
2. The patient never contradicts or denies to the doctor what I just reported the patient had said or done.
1. The patient does not have a callbell, does not call out "*NURSE, !!!!*", or demand that his unreasonable request be done because he was a physician in his old country.

Reprinted with permission. Retrieved June 6, 2005 from Emergency Nursing World Web site: www.ENW.org

What Does RN Really Stand For?
Nina Schroeder, RN
Richard Mintzer

Have you been confused about the meaning of RN since you finished becoming one? Do you find that other people think it actually means something other than what it does?

- Have you thought it might stand for *Really Nuts?*
- Do your patients think it stands for *Real Nice?*
- Does your head nurse think you're *Real Nervous?*
- Do doctors think it stands for *Right Now?*
- If you catch colds a lot does it stand for *Running Nose?*
- After twelve years of being overworked, does your therapist consider you *Really Neurotic?*
- Do nearsighted patients and ex-sailors think you're from the *Royal Navy?*
- After a long, hard day, are you sometimes mistaken for *Richard Nixon?*
- Do short people dislike you and does L.A. love you because they think you're *Randy Newman?*
- Does LPN also mean *Lousy Pay Nursing* or that you *Look Pretty Neat?*

From *The Unofficial Nurse's Handbook* by Nina Schroeder and Richard Mintzer, Copyright ©1986 by Ultra Communications, Inc. Used by permission of Dutton Signet, a division of Penguin Group (USA) Inc.

A Mind of ITs Own
Jane Bates

If women are from Venus and men from Mars, in that great space of conflicting notions that divides us is the Martian idea that computers 'do what you tell them.' Any Venusian knows this is not the case— computers have minds of their own. For instance, the other day I was typing in my department and the report printed out in A&E, which is at the other end of the hospital. This was 'my fault,' the IT (information technology) person said. Well, really.

One of the things that deters many nurses from returning to practice is the thought of all this new technology; the rumour has been spread that in hospitals nowadays 'it is all done by computers.' It is enough to send us off on a flight of fancy.

Would R2D2 lookalikes be gliding around the wards popping in thermometers and removing sutures with deft metallic fingers, while the nursing staff sit with their feet up eating chocolates? Come to think of it, that wouldn't put anyone off.

Computers in hospitals are nothing to be frightened of, even if they do bizarre things occasionally and leave you to carry the can. But getting used to them can seem like the final straw when there are so many other new things to learn. And do they really improve our lives?

I was an inpatient just before I came back to nursing and was fascinated by the amount of time the ward staff spent behind the desk hammering on the keyboard, their faces taut with concentration. Was this the shape of things to come, I wondered, or were they simply absorbed in an exciting game of *Tomb Raider?*

It is not surprising that people like me are wary of computers because, on the whole, they are not very encouraging. In fact, they eschew positive reinforcement altogether. They never say 'well done— you performed that cut and paste really well.' Rather, they starkly and randomly proclaim that you have 'performed an illegal operation,' which has you nervously looking over your shoulder and wondering whether or not to run for it.

Just like Martians, computers also have their own endearing eccentricities. In one place I worked, the computer had to be fanned regularly or it just shut down all on its own. Whatever human crisis was unfolding, someone had to keep waving a set of notes at the computer as though it were some kind of Eastern potentate. It somehow seemed symbolic of our reliance on the system and the necessity to keep it up and running at all costs. And it made you feel a right prawn if you were the one wielding the fan.

However we feel about it, IT is here to stay. Computers are an efficient tool for ordering and prescribing, for instance. Records can be accessed in a moment, providing a) you can remember your sign-in code, and b) that you can push in front of the ward clerk, house officer or whoever else is queuing up for the same terminal.

In our hospital the giving of medication is recorded on the computer system. There are no charts at the end of the beds for a weary house officer to scribble on and the nurses to puzzle over: 'If you hold it up this way it looks like she has written Frusemide, but in this light it looks like Occ. Chlor. It is 4 AM—should we phone and ask her?'

But I do miss the visible, tangible on-the-spot drug charts that are kept with the patients. It still seems safer to me. Why not adopt the belt and braces approach and have both?

If men are from Mars and women from Venus, then computers must be from the dark side of the moon. To most of us they are full of mystery yet they affect our lives in ways we do not even realise. And to ignore them would be sheer lunacy.

Reprinted with permission from Nursing Standard, ©2002; 16(35): 26.

Do You Know Me? I'm a Nurse

David J. Kearns, RN, MS

"Look! There's one of the doctors who put in the stitches when you hurt your hand," I heard a woman say to her three-year-old. As I maneuvered my way down the supermarket aisle, the boy and I eyed each other with suspicion. It was unlikely that I would forget him. He had nearly kicked me senseless before the doctor and I managed to restrain him.

"I'm a nurse," I said, smiling at his mother. "The other man was the doctor. He's the one who did the sewing."

"You're a nurse?"

"That's right."

"I've never met a male nurse before," she said. "You were wearing a white coat and you explained everything to me. I just assumed…"

"That's all right. I'm often mistaken for a physician."

Clothes Don't Always Make the Man

That mother's confusion was understandable. It's not easy to identify a man in nursing by what he wears. Sometimes I thumb through a catalog of uniforms that belongs to my wife, who is also a nurse. It contains less than one full page of items for men—mostly lab coats and zipper-front jackets. There's nothing specifically designed for a man in nursing.

It's just as bad in a uniform store, where I'll find only one rack of men's jackets and white, full-cut institutional trousers. That's not all. Everything I want is usually out of stock or has been discontinued by the manufacturer.

If I had chosen a career more traditional for my sex—airline pilot, construction worker, or truck driver—I wouldn't have these shopping problems. I'd know exactly what to wear. The locomotive engineer has his bib overalls and the rock singer his leather pants, but men in nursing are still searching for a unique, practical uniform that conveys a masculine identity.

When a woman dons a white uniform, she's easily recognized as a nurse. Put a white cap on her head, and there's no doubt about her identity. In fact, some hospitals require female nurses to wear caps for just that reason. Requiring me to observe a dress code, however, causes more identity problems than it solves.

A Male in White Spells Confusion

When I had to wear regulation whites, I was taken for a medical student, orderly, lab technician, dietary aide, housekeeper, and, on one notable occasion, a painter. Not even engraved name plates helped. On the other hand, if I wear anything other than white shirt, pants, and shoes, there are complaints that I might be mistaken for a physician.

Not having an easily recognizable uniform causes all kinds of problems with patients and supervisors. For one thing, the patient must go through a process of elimination to conclude that the man in white is a nurse. I can shorten the process by explaining again and again that I am, in fact, not an "intern or something,' but that wastes valuable nursing time.

Supervisors, too, have reacted strangely to my various outfits. Consider shoes, for example. If you want to know what it feels like to go surfing indoors, try running down a wet hospital hallway wearing a pair of men's clinic shoes. After sliding precariously while rushing blood samples to the lab, I decided to wear white leather athletic shoes with the logo of a popular manufacturer. I wore the shoes for a couple moths before any of my co-workers noticed them.

My supervisor, however, spotted my non-traditional footwear immediately. At my next evaluation, she rated my appearance as below standard because of my shoes. She expressed concern that one of the intubated, cannulated, drug-regulated patients in our ICU would peer over his bedrails, focus on my shoes, and suddenly feel unsure about the care he was getting.

Another supervisor objected to what she called "jogging shoes." I explained that half of my job did require jogging—around the ER and around the rest of the hospital for eight hours a night. She relented only after I challenged her to find a man's white shoe that would be comfortable while running, standing, pushing, and pulling. I was so convincing that she now wears running shoes herself.

How I Devised a Practical Solution

Since I now work in an ER without a rigid dress code, I've been able to devise an outfit I can recommend to other men in nursing. I located a line of khaki trousers that fit, wear well, and don't show blood too dramatically. The trousers, plus a white or tan polo shirt and a white, short-sleeved jacket comprise my outfit. On my belt, I carry my scissors, clamps, and penlight. I still wear jogging shoes, but they're tan colored and machine washable.

This wardrobe gives me comfort and flexibility. When I top off my outfit with stethoscope, pens, and note pads, I'm the well-dressed professional nurse ready to meet the public. When I take off my jacket, I'm ready for CPR, trauma, or dealing with an assaultive patient.

Perfect as my wardrobe may be, though, I'm still taken for a physician or an orderly. The world simply is not accustomed to a man in the nurse's role. This attitude will probably prevail until more men choose nursing as a career.

When that happens, a recognizable uniform for men will emerge. Until then, I'm thinking of ordering some new name plates. Printed before my name will be Real Nurse, Chief Pastry Chef, Mortician's Apprentice, or perhaps Rent This Space—just to see what happens.

Reprinted from RN, ©1986; 49(4): 63-64 with permission from the author.

I Wish I'd Shaved My Legs
Ged Cowin, RN, BEd

Last year I became a day surgery patient for a very simple gynaecological procedure—I feel I know you all well enough to say that now.

It started at about 8 AM. That man of mine very bravely sat with me in a waiting room with a dozen or so other women. He had one foot pointed towards the door and his fists were clenched ready to dash out the minute I gave him the sign that it was okay to go.

When I did, he started towards the door, slid to a halt, dashed back to peck me on the cheek and headed off to the lift without looking back.

I followed the girl who had called my name and was shown to a cubicle. 'Get undressed and pop this gown on,' were the instructions.

'Oh, the brochure said to bring my own dressing gown and slip-pers,' I said hopeful that I could wear my own.

'Nope, use this one, no slippers either.'

I look down begrudgingly at the bag of useless things that I had dragged in with me.

'Hmmm,' I wondered to myself, 'do I leave my underwear on or do I take it all off?" Now you might not think this matters, but when you are about to venture out to a public area with nothing but a gown on it matters a lot.

What if I take it all off and they are shocked. What if I leave it on and they laugh at me?

The gown was short—I wish I'd shaved my legs.

I poked my head out to ask for help. People everywhere but no one to help.

'Oh well, Ged old girl, go for broke,' I said, and took everything off.

So there I was, hairy legged, with just a threadbare piece of cotton between the world and my underworld.

A familiar face appeared. 'Okay follow me.' She didn't laugh thank goodness.

'Will my things be okay?" I asked? 'Yep.' She replied unconvinc-ingly. I glanced back at my bag of useless items and sighed.

I rounded a corner and entered a room with a sea of white gowns and bare legs. Young, old, fair, dark, we are all equal in the world of the waiting room.

But sensibly they all seemed to have socks on. I didn't think of that. By this time it was 10 AM. I sat on a chair and noticed one lady was knit-ting. She seemed to be here for the long haul.

One by one people were called, returned, were called again, returned again and were called a third and fourth time. I noticed after the fourth time they didn't come back.

I got nervous. Maybe there was a test and you couldn't get through until you knew the answer to some bizarre Monty Python type ques-tion about the wingspan of an African sparrow.

I was hysterical and pinched myself. It was the hunger affecting me. By now it was 12:30 PM. The knitting lady noticed the crazed look in my eyes. She told me they were a bit slow today.

I was called. I hoped they didn't ask me to count back from one hundred by sevens—I never could do that.

I was faced by my surgeon. Or so she said. She looked young, very young, very, very young.

'I have to ask you a few questions,' she said.

I looked around for the interview room. But she asked me right then and there in the passage, a thoroughfare with people going past, a cleaner leaning on a broom nearby. I was hesitant. Personal, intimate questions were thrown at me in a nonchalant matter. I tried to be worldly and grown up about it but I must say I was shocked.

My answers were somewhat guarded and I was sent back to the world of waiting once again.

Next time I was asked similar questions in the corridor by an anaesthetist, then it was back to the waiting room, and then a nurse came.

I couldn't help myself and asked her why the passageway? She apologised and found a quiet corner and actually offered me a chair.

I felt much better and poured my heart out to the poor girl.

'… and if only I'd known to bring socks,' I sobbed.

She looked tired. 'It'll be over soon,' she said, and sent me back to the world around the corner.

At last I was called for the fourth time. It was nearly 4 PM. I stood up resolutely, pulled my gown around me and marched forward to the operating suite. As I was led there, having drugs pushed into my arm, I noticed a room full of people, and thought 'Oh my God, they're all going to see me naked.' My last thoughts as I dozed off to sleep.

At 7 PM I was awake, sort of; dressed, sort of; fed, sort of; and, was offered a phone to ring that man of mine.

I called his mobile and imagined I could hear it ringing. It turned out I could. He was waiting right outside the recovery room for me, anxious.

He took my bag of useless items and gave me a hug. I cried for ages and ages. 'Crikey,' he said, 'what did they do to you?'

'Oh not much really,' I said and mumbled something about the wingspan of an African sparrow.

Reprinted with permission from Australian Nursing Journal, ©2002; 9(10): 40.

Bathroom Humor
Kathy Sitzman, BSN, RN

As a home care nurse working in what my employer refers to as an "outlying area," I cover a vast territory of both rural and urban settings. Due to a genetically predetermined condition called Miniature Bladder Syndrome, I have toiled to develop an intricate knowledge of public restrooms in my region. I thrill with the discovery of an easily accessible, nonrepulsive restroom.

Last week, I drove 60 miles to the main office for meetings. Road construction along the way led to frequent traffic backups. To pass away the time, I sang along with an oldies tape and sipped a rather large cup of iced tea. It would be an understatement to describe my condition as desperate as I approached the exit ramp at snail speed. Because I didn't see any restrooms between the exit and the office, I opted for the sure thing and sped toward the office amidst squealing tires and flying bags and clipboards.

Following a spectacular side-sliding entry into the parking lot, I bolted through the back door and ran straight for the ladies room. "I'll be with you in a minute," I called over my shoulder. The nurses I passed nodded knowingly in my direction.

After the meeting, I asked for advice on restrooms in the area. A crowd gathered and enthusiastically shared their data.

"Zeke's Gas-A-Teria is pretty clean but hard to find," said one.

"Lumpy's Fuel Emporium is on the main drag and has three stalls and a water fountain, but Old Lumpy gets mad if you use the john and don't buy gas," added another.

Another coworker commented, "Gloria's Gas-O-Rama is clean and right behind Dwayne's Donuts on First Street. Parking is a problem in the morning because of all the squad cars parked in front of the donut shop."

I made a mental note of these and other suggestions before hurrying away to another meeting. While at the meeting, I chuckled at the thought of creating a public restroom resource list. How useful this list would be to those of us who spend time on the road. Of course it would require a rating system. As the meeting droned on, the idea took root and grew.

Restroom Rating System

*Untidy Bowl: Potential health hazard; use only in an
    emergency
**The Uninvited Guest Rest: Toilet paper and soap usually
    available
***The Restroomer: Toilet paper and soap available; bug free;
    heated in winter.
****The Royale Flush: Includes all amenities featured in Restroomer;
    regular emptying of trash receptacles; hot running water;
    functional stall latches; spiffy décor.

A computer database listing all regional restrooms would follow. After that, a Web page (updated weekly) and a 24-hour hotline referred to as the Throne Phone.

What can I say? It was a long meeting and my imagination took over. However, if a hotline were available, I'd have the number programmed into my cellular phone's speed dial.

Reprinted with permission from Home Healthcare Nurse, ©1998; 16(11): 786.

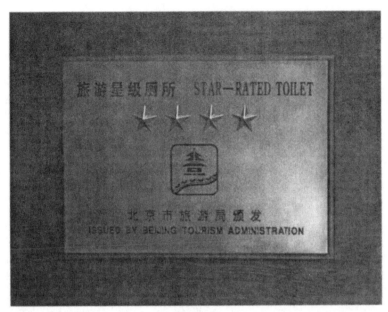

Four-star bathroom at Ming Tombs, Beijing, China (Photo by Kenneth Scott Young)

Yep, That's My Job Too!

David Powell, RN

Nursing demands that we be many things to many people, that we change roles as quickly as the average person changes hats, and that we be held responsible for each and every "hat" change we make. Here's an offbeat, upbeat view of our various areas of accountability.

According to Webster's Dictionary, accountability is "the state of being accountable, responsible, or liable." Fine. I joined the nursing profession with the knowledge that I'd be held accountable for my actions. I keep everything on the up and up. No liability here.

But where does my accountability for the care given a patient end and another professional's begin? At what point do I pass the buck? Harry Truman said, "The buck stops here." Was he referring to me and my other colleagues in nursing?

Based on my experience, the answer is Yes. Caring for long-term residents means that nursing and nurses are accountable for everything that happens in every minute of their day. Just when you think a patient's diet is the responsibility of the registered dietitian, a dietary aide asks you, "Can this patient have banana cream pie?" Well, can he?

Maybe, but is this patient diabetic? Is he IDDM or NIDDM? Is he permitted sweets beyond the norm for a diabetic? Should I check the patient's chart for this information, even though I'm feeding 30 other people at this very moment? Can I really stop him from eating what he wants to anyway?

Just how many hats am I expected to wear for this accountability thing?

No sooner do I administer this self-quiz than my attention is turned elsewhere: I receive explicit instructions that a certain postop skilled-care resident needs to start getting up to the bathroom to resume routine bowel movements. Unfortunately, on our first attempt, we find that the toilet is leaking. Now, it seems, my accountability as safety inspector takes over.

But wait, surely the maintenance department must be accountable here! After all, everyone's looking at me as if I can fix the toilet while the patient stands waiting. And what about getting a mop? Surely the mess needs to be mopped up before any further action can be taken. Isn't housekeeping accountable for that?

So, I delegate. The CNAs place the patient back in bed. A bedside commode is brought into the room. Housekeeping comes with the mop, eyeing nursing staff as idiots who can't even mop up a bit of water. Our maintenance man is called. He, too, is put out by the fact that nursing can't turn the toilet off and go elsewhere. Now he's got to fix it. Talk about accountability!

Leaving the room, the observant CNA notices ants crawling along the floorboard. What am I going to do about it? No way this patient can stay in a room infested with ants. The accountability bells start ringing again. Let me count the hats that are involved: exterminator, infection control, and entomologist for sure. After all, are these just ants or are they termites? Surely the nurse should know.

We move the patient to another room. Of course, a lot of charting must be done to account for the manner in which I handled the situation, demonstrating my accountability. It stands to reason that if I left the matter in the hands of those better equipped to fix it without explaining my own role and level of accountability, I would be held accountable for not being accountable.

As I chart, I suddenly notice I'm all alone on the ward. Where'd everybody go? Break time? Surely, they would have told me. After all, I'm accountable for their whereabouts. And, what about maintenance? Did they fix that toilet? Did housekeeping clean the room? Has somebody called the exterminator?

All right, I'll do it. It's my responsibility, somehow.

But, as I get started, a call light goes off. Here I go again. I am accountable for this; this is my department. Out of my way.

I answer the light of a sweet patient who has been with us a very long time. She wants to know how she looks today. Not in the clinical sense, but in the aesthetic sense. Is her hair combed nicely? Was her make-up put on correctly? Do her clothes match?

The hair stylist, the fashion designer, and the therapist hats go on. I dole out praises worthy of Casanova, stopping just short of flattery that might constitute behavior for which I wouldn't want to be held accountable. She is appeased. But wait...

Her sweet tooth is acting up. Could I get her something from the vending machine in the break room? Certainly. I slap on the delivery boy's hat.

She wants a Twix Bar, but if they don't have Twix, get a Milky Way, and if no Milky Way, then Three Musketeers will do. If not that, then M&Ms—not the ones with peanuts, her dentures won't tolerate peanuts. And, she doesn't like the red ones, either; she still thinks they cause cancer. Should I tell her what the green ones do?

I go to the break room, where I find all my staff. Should I mention my accountability for them leaving the floor without telling me? Maybe later, when I can get each one alone. No sense tackling a gang.

I look at my left hand where I wrote down all the instructions for my delivery boy job. On my right hand I've scribbled doctor's orders for a new prescription for another resident, reminding me of my nursing role (yes, it does arise from time to time). What to do, what to do? I hope I don't mix them up. I'd really be accountable for that!

Okay, no Twix Bar. But there is a Milky Way! I make the purchase and deliver the merchandise as instructed. Now, to finish charting and write that order, not forgetting the five other orders I need to write. My accountability is nearing its close. If I can just sit down for a few minutes and chart while everyone else accounts for their responsibilities, I'd be thrilled. But wait...

The dentures of another patient will not fit properly. Okay, the dentist hat goes on. And another resident needs his toenails cut, while another wants her fingernails trimmed. Put on those podiatrist and manicurist hats. Don't forget that the brace in room 12 needs adjusting, the resident's family in room 6 wants to speak with me, the air conditioning in room 2 is blowing hot air, there's some wallpaper hanging down in room 4, and the lights in room 5 keep turning on and off. Get the physical therapist, family counselor, environmental control, interior decorator, and electrician hats out!

Have I missed anything? I'm sure I have. Probably a million other hats we wear every day as nurses.

It's funny, though; I wouldn't have it any other way. All of these hats are additional burdens, to be sure. But, at the same time, I feel proud that no task is too small when it comes to the health and comfort of my patients.

Besides, who better to keep up with patient needs than the RN in charge? Who better to advocate for patient care? Who better than the one professional who remains with the patient while others come and go? Nursing is 24-hour care.

So, grumble a bit, bite your lip, gnash your teeth. But, get up and check that toilet, the wallpaper, and the lights. Tell others to do the same. Then check that they have checked.

Wear your accountability like a badge. Take charge and just do it. After all, no one else is going to.

Reprinted from RN, ©2000; 63(2): 41-42 with permission from the author.

Images of The Perfect Nurse
T. Pursley

- Gives all enemas and suppositories at the beginning of her shift.
- Tapes report in three minutes flat.
- Volunteers to float to another unit when it's your turn.
- Never complains about the schedule, doctors, nurse/patient ratios, administrators, excessive paperwork, other shifts. Never complains.
- Keeps meticulous documentation to satisfy insurance companies, attorneys, DEHEC and the JCAHO.
- Never calls a Doctor past 9 PM. Ever.
- Understands all physician mumbling and handwriting.
- Is available to give massages, manicures, pedicures and facials.
- Knows the exact time the doctor will be making rounds.
- Responds to call lights immediately, with pain medicine in hand.

Those that try to be the 'perfect nurse' most often succumb to the pressure by:
- Burning out.
- Leaving nursing.
- Taking respite in alcohol, drugs or a locked ward.

Good Nurses, give the best care they can to each patient, within the time they have. Then these Good Nurses go home to:
- Devour a half-gallon of chocolate-chocolate chip ice cream with hot fudge and nuts.
- Soak in a hot tub.

Reprinted with permission from Journal of Nursing Jocularity, ©1995; 5(1): 20-21. Edited from the original.

Paydirt
Paula J. Wilshe, BA

One early morning this week, our department manager, Kathie, breezed into the registration area to collect the ED charts from the day before. She turned, smiled, and, almost as an afterthought, said,

"When the inside secretary gets here we'd like her to watch the window while you come back to the office and start learning to do the payroll." There was nothing in her expression that indicated the morning's business would be any more taxing than a cozy chat with coffee, some shared pleasantries, and oh, let's write down the names of everyone who worked yesterday.

"Sure," I said, enthusiastically, eager to broaden my knowledge base, facilitate my personal growth, and demonstrate to my boss that I am ever eager to please. Because she writes my yearly evaluations, I believe it is prudent to do so on an occasional basis.

My original understanding of the task was that people worked, and you paid them. I thought "doing the payroll" was simply a catch phrase for walking to the cashier's office every other Friday to pick up the departmental paychecks. I did not consider the possibility that math skills might be involved.

Judy had set out an impressive array of computer printouts, sharpened pencils (both black and red), rulers, and about 50 laminated cheat sheets detailing employee numbers, shifts, vacation requirements, codes for their reimbursement, their favorite colors, and whether they had ever been guilty of departmental insubordination or had been involved in any sort of fracas in the nurses' station. "These are the tools we use," she said, "to determine the final paycheck."

I began to feel nervous. "Kathie," I said, through the open door to her office, "Did I ever tell you that I have two checking accounts?"

"No, you didn't," she answered pleasantly. "That's nice."

"I have a green one and a blue one," I continued quickly. "Because I don't know how to balance them, so I use one until it gets a little hot, then I use the other one while the first one cools down."

Kathie and Judy burst into bubbling laughter. "I told you she was really funny," Judy said. "Isn't she funny? She always makes me laugh."

I picked up a pencil and tried to focus on one of the computer printouts. There were names and numbers and codes and clock-in times and clock-out times and all of them were swimming around on the page.

"It's really very simple," said Judy, "everyone gets paid straight time which is a number 1, unless they worked overtime, or did not take a lunch break, which would be a number 2. You really have to watch that, though, because some people get paid overtime if they work more than 8 hours in a day, and some people get paid overtime only if they work more than 40 hours in a week, or 80 hours in a pay period. It all depends on which waiver they've signed, so you always have to check to see if they're an 8-, 12-, or 40-hour employee. That's also dependent on whether or not the month begins with a J, and if a full moon occurs at any time during the pay period. You can always refer to this chart here. If they took a vacation day, that's a number 15, but if it was a vacation/sick day, that's a number 20, unless it was their second sick day, and that's a number 483. Of course, the holidays are a number 32 if they worked, but are a number 33 if they weren't scheduled to work the holiday but it was their normal day to work, but they don't get a weekend or shift differential on the holiday bonus. If they didn't work but have depleted their vacation time, you give them a code 11 and 2 hours of detention, and if they didn't sign the exception sheet they don't get paid at all. If they traded shifts you have to adjust their shift differential accordingly, and always remember to add in the week-end diff. If they worked but they didn't do a good job, you can write "delete" over their names. You have to bear in mind that night shift's holidays and weekends are actually the night *before* the holiday, and in any case, of course, we differentiate between the shifts by placing an S1, S2, or S3 beside their tallies, except for Claudia who works 1 to 9 but gets paid straight second shift, and Mary who works 10:30 to 7:00 but gets paid first shift for her first 4 hours, and second shift for her second 4 hours. Unless she works overtime, of course." She handed me the red pencil. "Now you do it."

At that moment Claudia came through the door to tell Kathie that a visiting physician had hurled the urology cart into the med room in a fit of pique and that some of the more timid nurses were barricaded in the dictation room.

"Look, Claudia," I said, with a weak smile, "I'm doing the payroll."

"That's nice, sweetie," she said, squeezing my shoulder. She walked into Kathie's office, and as she pulled the door shut behind her I thought I heard her say tensely, "Kathie, you are aware, are you not, that she has two checking accounts, a green one and a blue one..."

I looked down at the computer printout and decided to start with Claudia's name because I'm familiar with her hours, her shift, and I know her employee number by heart. "Let's see," I murmured," 8 hours of straight time, second shift, no overtime," I made a few notations on the paper. I pushed it across the desk to Judy.

Judy stared at it for a few moments before speaking. "I realize you do most of the ED billing," she said kindly, "but instead of paying Claudia for her shift yesterday you have charged her for an Established Patient Low Complexity and an 18 French catheter."

"Oh," I said. "I'll try it again."

That pretty much sums up how the week has been. I have gotten to the point where I can do the daily printouts without help, and I have somehow gotten through the painful process of the "weekly run," a horror better left unexplored. Judy has been very patient, and Claudia has been sweet and solicitous. Kathie gave me a Tootsie Pop and told me I was a nice girl when the inside secretary screamed at me for taking too long in the office.

Next Friday is payday, and I am hoping that all the numbers I carefully documented will come out in correct monetary issue when the checks are finally printed. Me, I'm not too worried. My paycheck is direct-deposited into my green account, and we are using the blue one this week.

What are YOU Like?

Jane Tyke

Are you cut out for the perils of practice nursing or perhaps you have missed your vocation in the Peace Corps? Are you a paragon of virtue or would you benefit from a visit to charm school? Are you ruthless or spineless? I've devised this personality test to help you uncover the real you.

1. It's Friday lunchtime and you are running late. Your last two patients are departing for a world trip in 2 days and request all the vaccinations that the travel agent advocated. Do you:
   a. Stick in loads of needles then cheerfully announce that they won't be effective in time and recommend good travel insurance.
   b. Sigh and kiss your lunch goodbye. Then spend the next hour giving thorough, evidence-based travel advice, obtaining informed consent, administering vaccines, documenting everything meticulously, and generating the IOS claims that pay your wages.
   c. Commiserate that they have left it too late and direct them to the nearest BA Travel Clinic.
   d. Ask if they need someone to carry their suitcases while grabbing your free samples of sunscreen and insect repellant.
2. A notorious, frequent attender marches up to the reception desk. She insists that her child needs antibiotics again as she's "just not herself at all." Little Shakira-Jade is meanwhile running amok and redecorating the waiting room with her breakfast crips and cola. How would you deal with this challenging situation?
   a. Immediately refer her to your favourite GP. You have no paediatric training and you can't be too careful with ill kids can you?
   b. Thoroughly examine the child, then firmly but gently explain the latest research on unnecessary antibiotics and give appropriate advice.

    c. Watch in awe as Shakira-Jade wreaks havoc and imagine what it is like when she is herself. Then get rid of her with a prescription like the doctor usually does.

    d. Congratulate Mum on her parenting skills to gain her trust. Then—never missing an opportunity to promote health—give her a leaflet on healthy eating along with the scrip.

3. There is a baby-faced drugs rep lurking in the waiting area. Naturally the doctors have all fled, so the receptionist has kindly granted him an audience with you instead. While he recites his piece about the latest miracle cure, do you:

    a. Impishly challenge the poor dolt on the validity of the trials he is quoting. His business card may boast "BA (Hons)" but it's probably in film studies anyway.

    b. Glaze over while managing to look interested, and mentally review this week's shopping.

    c. Let him finish his spiel then trill: "Sorry, I don't do asthma," pick up your shopping list and prepare to do battle at Tesco.

    d. Inform him you are about to become a nurse prescriber in the hope of getting some decent freebies for a change instead of sticky pads and pens.

4. The rep thanks you for your precious time and shows his gratitude by leaving a few sticky pads and pens. How do you react?

    a. Go and let the tyres down on his BMW. A mere whippersnapper should not be in charge of such a dangerous toy.

    b. Thank him graciously, for we always need sticky pads and pens

    c. Contemplate exactly where he can stick his post-its.

    d. Alert security to block the exits until he hands over a snazzy car cleaning kit like the doctors get.

5. One of the GPs regularly nabs you for something just as you are getting ready for home. Tonight, it's a four-layer dressing. Do you:

    a. Look genuinely crestfallen as you explain that it's assertiveness training night. Then hand over the dressings and wish him luck.

    b. Humbly remove your coat and get on with it. There's nothing on telly tonight anyway.

    c. Do the darned dressing as quickly as possible then refer the patient to the district nurses, the wound care experts (you might just catch EastEnders).

    d. Politely point out that you are merely a wage-slave and not a profit-sharing partner and demand some recompense.

6. A family of four scheduled for new patient interviews have not turned up, leaving you with some rare free time. How would you spend it?

    a. Stick the kettle on, put your feet up and tackle those unopened *Practice Nurse* magazines

b. Help your colleague with her list of patients
c. Tidy out the sluice, some habits die hard
d. Knock off early—you're owed loads of overtime from Dr Pest!

So what do your answers reveal about you?

Mostly (a) You have a wicked streak in you but it's probably just
    your coping mechanism.
Mostly (b) Professional to the core, what an inspiration to us all!
Mostly (c) A bit of a martyr sometimes, but can also be pushed
    too far.
Mostly (d) On the ball, sharp as a knife, you never miss a trick.
A complete mixture? Evidently, you are multi-faceted and can react
unpredictably. Generally speaking professional and reliable, you can
put up with most things but are not a complete pushover. You can
stand up for yourself and sometimes use attack as the best form of
defence. You should do well in practice nursing!

Reprinted with permission from Practice Nurse, ©2004; 28(1): 50-51.

'Twas the Night Before Christmas
Kathy Payton, LPN, MT

'Twas the night before Christmas all through ICU,
The patients were restless, the nurses were too.
The IVs were hung on their IMEDs in rows,
The patients assessed from their heads to their toes.

While Ruth who's still nesting and I took a break,
Paul made some coffee for hot caffeine's sake.
When out in the hall there arose such a clatter,
We sprang from our chairs to see what was the matter.

The florescent lights cast a glare on the floor,
As we scrambled and squeezed to get through the door.
Then what to our wondering eyes should appear,
But three ER nurses with a bed full of cheer.

The patient was gasping and breathing his last,
So we called Dr. Parker and said, "Make it fast."
As leaves that before a wild hurricane blew,
We flew in the unit and called out, "Code Blue!"

More rapid than eagles, he was moved from the cart,
The nurses and others, we all did our part.
On Pamela, Steven, Paula, Donna and Sue,
June, Becky and Becky, and Charles, you too!

The Patient needs oxygen, he's blue and then green,
This is the weirdest thing we've ever seen.
And then in a twinkling we heard from the bed,
"What are you doing? You'd think I was dead!"

We jumped in surprise, then we laughed and shook hands,
Sat down and waited for enzymes and bands.
Shelly and Mary were listing his loot,
His clothes trimmed with fur, his left and right boot.

He asked us to check on the rooftop in back,
For some valuable animals and a great big red sack.
His eyes were now twinkling, his breathing was steady,
His color was better, he said, "Now I am ready."

We tried to instruct him about AMA,
He stubbornly said, "I must be on my way."
He put his old pipe in his bow of a mouth,
"Now I must get headed north, east, west, and south."

Dear Santa, we pleaded, won't you let us try,
To help you get over your stroke or MI?"
He winked at the gang and he twisted his head,
And promised us that we had nothing to dread.

The night was near over and he had to work,
So he gave us our stockings and turned with a jerk.
He blew a shrill whistle, his team came so quick,
Then flash out the window went good old St. Nick.

He sprang to his sleigh to his team gave a whistle,
His last words to us floated down like a thistle,
"Don't worry dear children, it's not my lungs or heart,
These dang deer ate Mexican, man do they fart!"

Reprinted with permission from Journal of Nursing Jocularity, ©1996; 6(4): 10-11.

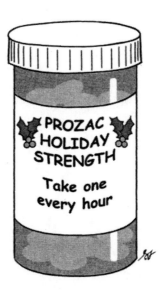

'Twas the Night..."
Linda Snyder, RN, MSN, CRNP, CEN

'Twas the night before Christmas, when all through the ED

The nurses were waiting for what was to be.

IVs were hung by the bedsides with care

For the traumas and MIs that soon would be there.

The charts were nestled all snug in their slots

While med students practiced with sutures and knots.

And the staff in their scrubs with nary a cap,

Thought how nice it would be to just take a nap

When out on the drive there arose such a clatter,

We sprang from the desk to see what was the matter.

Away to the doors we flew like a flash,

We watched intently, it felt sort of like M*A*S*H.

The voice on the console of the radio below

Gave us more info than we needed to know.

When what to my wondering eyes should appear

But an ambulance loaded with Santa and reindeer.

The EMT driver, so lively and quick,

Had been summoned on 9-1-1 by St Nick.

The response had been rapid, the medics they came

As Santa had listed each reindeer by name.

Dasher had mono, Dancer had flu, Prancer was limping and Vixen was too.

Comet had migraines, Cupid felt punk, Donder was listless and Blitzen was drunk.

From the front door at triage to the treatment room walls

Was heard the call, "Treat them fast! Cure them all!"

As the nurses who work in the ED all know,

Reindeers oft think that the service is slow.

So up to the patients the nurses all flew

With IVs and meds and compassion too.

And then in a twinkling I heard on the roof

The whirring of a chopper, not reindeer hoofs.

As I drew in my head, and was turning around,

Through the metal detector St Nicholas came with a bound.

He was dressed all in fur from his head to his foot,

And his clothes were all tarnished with ashes and soot.

The questions on insurance had him confused.

Which PCP had the reindeer all used?

His eyes how they twinkled! His dimples how merry!

Everyone noticed, though they were all in a hurry.

His droll little mouth was drawn up like a bow,

As he worried about toys and the kids and the snow.

The stump of the pipe he held tight in this teeth,

Couldn't provide smoke to encircle his head like a wreath.

He'd been told several times that he couldn't smoke,

So he settled for microwave popcorn and Coke.

The reindeer were better, feeling stronger and well.

Boy, would they have a story to tell.

The winks of their eyes and twists of their heads

Soon gave Santa to know he had nothing to dread.

The staff spoke not a word, but went straight to their work,

Completing the charts, then turned with a jerk

And giving each reindeer instructions on care,

Reminded them all that "We're always there!"

The deer sprang to their sleigh, St Clause gave a whistle,

And away they all flew like the down of a thistle.

But we heard him exclaim, ere he drove out of sight,

"You are Angels of Christmas! Have a good night!"

Reprinted from Journal of Emergency Nursing, ©1998; 24(6): 482 with permission from The Emergency Nurses Association.

The Road You Didn't Take

Each of us has tailored our education and designed our life and career exactly the way we want it and, hopefully, living it. It probably means having taken a great leap of faith in ourselves—in our skills, abilities, diligence, strength of purpose, and our own persistence. It is important that we believe in something, anything, and spend each and every day refusing to fail. Insist on success on your own terms, and nobody else's.

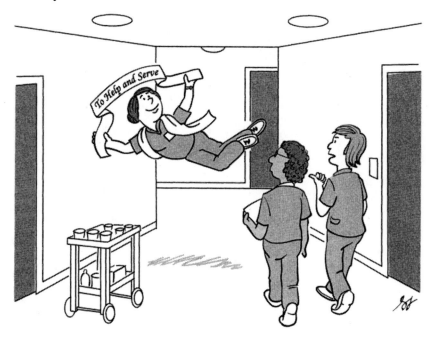

Nursing student.

Professor Plume's Letters
Patricia Plume

Dear Nursing Times,
  A week ago I sent you copies of my research paper entitled: 'Meta-research: a qualitative analysis of researchers' attitude to research.'

While not expecting you to understand it I did expect you to recognise, via my qualifications and standing in the world of nursing research, the implicit worth of the paper. But I came down to breakfast this morning to discover a letter from your journal telling me that you have sent my article out for peer review.

Let's assume for a moment that you would recognise my peers if one of them fell on you in some kind of bizarre charity parachute-jump accident, and let's assume that you had by some strange illicit way learned where they live, I wonder what you might hope to achieve by asking them to review my work?

As the great French philosopher René Descartes said: 'I think therefore I am.' I'm sure she would not mind me paraphrasing her work when I say: 'I wrote it and therefore it is.' If someone with my academic prowess does a piece of work you can rest assured it is a good piece of work. They don't just give out professorships with reward points at the local supermarket, you know.

I came close to withdrawing my paper. If I had wanted a peer review I would subject it to the highly esteemed and exclusively read *Journal of Venerable Nursing Research*, where I know my work will be rigorously reviewed by a very good friend. However, my fiancé Patrick, who has been a tower of strength throughout my academic rise, convinced me that it was time to, as he so shrewdly put it, 'broaden my appeal.'

He said I should think of myself as the nursing research equivalent of Pavarotti. Most of my work is for a knowing and distinguished audience engaged with high culture but occasionally, in the interests of charity or at least the greater good, I should be prepared to duet with U2. So I have chosen not to withdraw the paper, but you have Patrick to thank for that.

Before signing off I couldn't help but notice your news story concerning the NMC finding a £7m shortfall in its pension fund. This seems likely to result in a registration fee increase. While I realise this may anger some nurses and embarrass the relatively new but oft-embarrassed NMC, I wonder if a little academic perspective on this issue might be of use.

Research has shown that if one pays more for say, an item of jewellery, it is treated as more valuable. I wonder if the same might not apply to registering as a nurse. If nurses have to pay more in order to practise might they not logically come to value themselves more highly? I believe this is a theory worth testing and look forward to setting up a randomised controlled trial soon after the NMC announces that it intends to recover its investment losses directly from nurses.

If you'd like to sponsor this research I would offer you first publication rights. The Americans refer to this as a 'win-win situation.' The NMC gets its money, I get funding for research, you get first publication rights to seminal research and nurses get to feel good about the fact that nursing is more expensive and thus of greater value to them. Like I said, they don't give out professorships for nothing.

Yours sincerely,
Professor Patricia Plume

My Most Humorous Moment in Nursing
Eva L. Knab

To me, the zealous but apprehensive nursing student, the med room was a place of mystery where only the chosen dared enter. Inside were walls of forbidden cabinets closely guarding their neat little rows of bottles and boxes of all sizes. Here was stored all those wonderful medications with the outrageously complicated names I had been struggling to become familiar with. It was a very small room whose counter was laden with little family groups of cups and rolls of tape and goodies of all sorts. Lining the counters' back wall were the injection syringes, appearing to be regally guarding the kingdom above and around them, all buttoned up tight in their many colored jackets. From this sanctuary would come forth the many tablets and capsules, and the elixirs and powders the world of pharmacology had prepared to ease the pain and suffering of our patients. It was one of those innocent little powders that would sorely try my soul this day.

What an exciting day this was for me! How much I had looked forward to passing meds and, oh my, what were those little feathers doing, prancing around inside of my stomach? I knew I could only give the simplest of medicines today, but here I was almost a real nurse, full of hope and impatience to begin this new role. I had reviewed and prepared myself with much gusto and felt a great surge of confidence, totally disregarding the behavior of my stomach.

After being soundly oriented and introduced to the inhabitants of the room, I was given my med assignments and at last was on my own and ready to conquer the day. As I had been so well taught, I thoroughly checked and rechecked my orders and the medication, reading the symbols and instructions with great care. I selected the baby and her six-ounce brother from the cup family on the counter and set to work. The medicine was a gritty looking powder to be mixed with six ounces of water. I measured as carefully as if I were mixing volatile chemicals in that tiny cup and when I was sure it was right, poured the powder into the water. Finding the stir sticks among the treasures on the counter, I began to mix as I picked up my orders for the big moment. Back went my shoulders and up went my chin as I boldly sallied forth to deliver my potion to the patient down the hall.

As I neared the designated door, I gave the mixture another stir or two to keep it from separating. "Yuck, I thought, this stuff sure looks gooey. I'd hate to have to swallow it!" With every step the cup seemed to be more filled, and I thought it looked strange. At the doorway, I knocked, and a little squeaky voice said, "Come in," so taking a big breath, I went in. There on the bed was this wizened little lady looking for all the world like a little pixie in her pink ruffly bed jacket. I re-read the orders once again and greeted my little patient as I checked her arm band to avoid any error, while my eyes kept being drawn to the cup of "whatever" in my hand. Deciding that this would take a lot of water to wash down, I placed the cup on the table and filled the pitcher while wondering how in the world this little lady would swallow whatever I had to offer her. Still undaunted, I picked the cup back up and tried to stir it again for good measure, but the stick would barely move! The cup no longer held a mixture, but a stiff, gooey brown mass that was apparently alive and trying to climb out of its prison.

I looked at my patient and she was staring at the cup in disbelief. In a voice that set me back on my feet she screeched, "You want me to drink that stuff?" For me this was one of those "please earth, open up and swallow me" moments. I wished I could just disappear. I must have garbled something of an excuse, I don't know what, but somehow it got me out the door. I don't know how long I stared at this monster I had created, but my mind was sure working overtime. I thought about this movie I had seen where this "blob" couldn't be destroyed and as it grew, it simply enveloped everyone and everything in its way. Here I was holding my own personal blob and it was about to phagocytize me! By this time it was up over the top of the cup like a gross, brown ice cream. Maybe I could flush it down the toilet, but no, it would surely clog the drain and the whole hospital would be flooded! I knew I had to face the music, to take it back to the room of mystery where it was born. I couldn't even think about what my instructor would do when she saw this "thing that was growing right in my hands!"

As I recall, the walk back to my fate took at least half a lifetime. As I passed each doorway, I dreaded that perhaps one of my fellow students would come out at that very moment and catch me in the act of whatever it was I was doing wrong. Worst of all, I had to pass the nurses' station where all the RNs would see me, nurses who had certainly never done anything so absurd as this. By the time I entered the med room, I was holding my prize out at arms' length with both hands as if it were a bomb about to explode. It was over the sides and oozing over my fingers and all I wanted at that moment was to get rid of it.

My instructor had the most memorable incredulous look on her face as she watched me, and all I could say was, "Something's not quite right here." Then, heaven must have opened because I heard the voice of an angel saying, "Just toss it in the trash, right over there in the corner." And I did just that, separating myself from this nemesis as quickly as possible. As I went back to my instructor, I saw that she had turned her head away from me. I thought "this is it, my career has ended. I'm all done." She grasped her stomach and I was sure the "blob" had sickened her to the point of vomiting. When an eternity had passed and she finally looked at me, I saw tears streaming down her face and she was laughing! When I realized she wasn't upset I began to laugh too, a little, but my tears were from relief, not humor. Strangely, through my tears, a new feeling began to come over me, a sort of warmth. As I looked around that little room I had so dreaded, it became my haven. I loved every corner, every gorgeous cabinet with all the terrific little supplies. Everything in there became my friend. I would be back to try again! Wow! Life was great! I laughed then, from deep down, even though I still wasn't sure what was so funny.

When we were able to settle down and exhibit some measure of control, we reviewed the orders and scrutinized the package of the guilty powder. The secret was found to be in the way the order was written. What should have been a dram with its little z-like squiggly with a tail, had been written as an ounce with two little squiggles and a tail! That dear little lady down the hall had almost been offered eight times the intended volume of the fiber preparation.

Since that day, my instructor has often used the incident as an example of confusing orders and I have not hesitated to question anything that didn't seem right. Every time I stir that mixture, I remember my "blob" and smile a secret smile.

Reprinted from Imprint, Vol. 40, Number 4, Sept/Oct 1993, ©National Student Nurses' Association, Inc.

Constipation Among Operating Room Nurses: Flatulence as Evidence

Dr. Kant Go, RN (alias Dennis Ross, RN, MAE, PhD)

Purpose of the Proposed Study

The purpose of this proposed study is to identify the incidence of constipation among members of the surgical team and to correlate this incidence with the rate of flatulence per surgical team member during surgery lasting longer than 3 hours.

The Research Problem

Introduction of noxious fumes to the surgical area may be associated with:

1. Prolonged length of surgery as the surgeon takes time to look for potential bowel perforation or bowel incontinence
2. Distraction from the surgery by one or more members of the team (as directly related to the duration and concentration of the noxious release); and
3. Physical findings of nausea, paleness, strabismus, rhinorrhea, or shortness of breath experienced by proximate members of the surgical team.

Significance of the Proposed Study

This study will provide significant information on the noxious odors that occasionally invade the surgical area, even when bowel surgery is not being performed. However, when bowel surgery is being performed, this phenomenon is of especial concern because of the often-erroneous conclusion that the bowel has inadvertently been entered.

Research Questions

The research questions that will guide this study are:

1. Is there a relationship between the incidence of constipation among members of the surgical team and the length of surgery and associated physical complaints of the surgical team in surgical procedures lasting longer than 3 hours?
2. Is there a relationship between the incidence of diet (especially intake of bran, brussel sprouts, baked beans, cabbage, wild leek soup,* and similar flatulogenic foods) of the surgical team and the length of surgery or physical complaints during surgery?
3. Is there a relationship between the obnoxiousness of the odor and the degree of constipation?

Theoretical Framework

The theoretical framework used to design the study and within which the study results will be interpreted is Pee-Yew's corollary on gas movements. Enough said about that.

Design

A double-blind (either already blind or purposely blinded for this study) and double non-blind descriptive design will be used.

---

*Dr. I.M. Obnoxious reported in the July 1876 *Anals of Medicine* that wild leek soup has been used by certain performers on the West Bank of Paris to produce excessively long episodes of flatulence (some reported as long as 307 seconds), which were used to accomplish a sort of music.

Method

Sample

A purposive (not explosive) stratified sampling methodology will be used to include both rural and urban medical centers with surgery suites containing 2 to 12 ORs. Only surgeries planned to last longer than 3 hours will be used (permitting adequate accumulation of flatulence to ensure its necessary release during the procedure). Operating Rooms using individualized closed scrub suits with personalized air flow will not be included in the sample (mainly because the operator does not affect other members of the OR team and must stand, or perhaps sit, in his or her own pew).

Data Collection

Two blind and two nonblinded data collectors will be used to collect data. The blind data collectors will identify the source of flatulence to within one person on either side of the flatulee (releaser of flatulence). Once the general area of the flatulee has been identified, the nonblinded data collectors will use the Supernumerary Noxious Inhalant Filter (SNIFer) to identify the actual source of the flatulence. Once the source is identified, one nonblinded data collector will then use the supersensitive SNIFer to identify any subsequent flatulee releases. When subsequent releases are identified, the second nonblinded data collector will time the length of release and determine the severity of obnoxiousness using the Degree of Observable Obnoxiousness (DOO) scale (each incident thereafter recorded as a DOO incident). After each surgical procedure, the blind observers will retain the flatulee while the nonblinded observers collect information on the flatulee's normal, or abnormal, bowel elimination patterns.

Instruments

1. Supernumerary Noxious Inhalant Filter (SNIFer): (Odious, 1984) has shown reliability and validity in the identification of flatulees in a wide variety of settings and circumstances. This instrument is recalibrated before each use with specially prepared test tubes containing standard measures of obnoxious odors.
2. The Degree of Observable Obnoxiousness (DOO) scale: The DOO scale is an investigator-developed instrument that uses observable (paleness, strabismus, rhinorrhea) and reportable (nausea) parameters to identify the degree of obnoxiousness associated with the odor as determined by the proximate members of the operating team.

Data Anal-Ysis

All data will be coded (and filtered to reduce malfunction of the data analyzers and computers) and entered into computers. Multiple regression and ego regression will be used for statistical analysis, using the Correlation Regression Analysis Program (CRAP).

Limitations

The results of this study will obviously be confined to the population of OR teams, in which the problem is so rampant (thank goodness).

Future Research

Having identified the prevalence of this problem, the investigator plans to develop experimental studies of interventions designed to specifically counteract the problem. Such interventions might include placing odor mufflers in flatulees, provision for enemata before procedures longer than 3 hours for repeater flatulees, and use of Flatulent Arrest or Retardant Traps (FARTs) for flatulees.

Funding

Funding resources will need to be further explored, but it is assumed that the recipients of the flatulee's expressions of constipation will see this as a useful and rewarding project and gladly donate large sums of money to accomplish this much-needed research.

References

Doubting-Thomas A: Can these fecoliths actually represent the size of brontosaurus constipated stools? You bet! Scatology for Beginners 42:24-32, 1995.

Gas X: Don't blame us! Anals of Anesthesia 14:34-39, 1995.

Go K: What is this thing called... constipation? Anals of Medicine 32:54-59, 1992.

Gross IM, Odour HS: Symptoms associated with constipation: "Doc it hurts and I can't go!" Current Issues in the Anorectum 14:56-59, 1985.

Jong E: Flubberblasters and SBD's: Morbidity in sexual partners. Fear of Farting 2:45-49, 1982.

National Institute for Nursing: Let's find out about outcomes: Ask every patient about their BMs. Annual Report of the NIN, 1993, pp 2-4.

National Institute for Nursing: Ever hear about outcomes? Let's pay more attention to patients' BMs. Annual Report of the NIN, 1994, pp 3-4.

National Institute for Nursing: Come on, this is important stuff: Pay more attention to patients' BMs. Annual Report of the NIN, 1995, pp 13-14.

National Institute for Nursing: You think we're kidding? You'd best pay more attention to patients' BMs. Annual Report of the NIN, 1996, pp 43-44.

National Institute for Nursing: Oh, come on, PLEASE: Pay more attention to patients' BMs. Annual Report of the NIN, 1997, pp 73-74.

National Institute for Nursing: Rates of terminal constipation linked to nurses' avoidance behaviors. Annual Report of the NIN, 1998, pp 100-104.

Nosier SS: Epidemic laboratory rat deaths linked to constipated laboratory attendant: The cost of science to wild life. New York Times: Science Section, April 1, 1985, p 34.

Seymour-Pitts TT: What exemplifies outcomes research more than the outcomes of constipation? (Editorial). Views From the Rectum: Endoscopy Made Easy 2:12, 1995.

Tremors E: Measuring free gas levels in the OR: Serendipitous findings. Anesthesiology and the Common Man 14:3-7, 1990.

Urp B: Noxious airs: Flatulence as a social enigma? Journal of Ephemeris Sociology 4:34-45, 1984.

Willy W, Peter P: The prevalence of constipation among OR staff: Support for Freud's speculations on anal retentiveness? Psychomorphic Psychology 12:24-34, 1991.

Wilting IM: Is all that gas in the OR related to anesthesia: Hell no! OR Supervisor 12:23-25, 1994.

Yew P: Is the gas dense or are YOU?! Chapter 4, in Gaseous Corollaries to Denseness: How Thick Is It? Buttsfield, NJ, Butts' Better Press, 1990.

Reprinted from Seminars in Perioperative Nursing, ©1999; 8(2): 85-87 with permission from Elsevier.

Do Your Own Homework
Rita J. Lourie, RN

At a large medical center in Boston, Mass., a young nursing student was giving an elderly patient an extensive examination. After asking her to name the presidents backwards, he said, "Now I want you to help me with some math problems."

Frustrated, the woman said, "Now listen, Sonny. You probably went to Harvard, and all your friends probably went to Harvard. Have *them* help you with your math."

Reprinted with permission from Journal of Nursing Jocularity.

Pie-eyed and Deskless

Nick Hinchliffe

I have just had my annual—for the first time in three years—moving and handling and basic life support study day. I confess I wasn't looking forward to going, but in the end I found it an interesting exercise, not least in staying awake.

I am one of those people who has to fight to keep my eyes open when sat in a classroom, regardless of the time of day or the subject being discussed. When I begin to get a little heavy about the eyelids, I try to disguise it by shielding my eyes in what I hope appears to be a thoughtful pose, or I slouch over the desk if there is one. (My number one complaint about nurse education at the moment is these 'open classroom' arrangements—no desk equals nowhere to sleep.)

But all this subterfuge is wasted when, just as I nod off, I jerk awake with a grunt to reveal my cheek shiny with drool. This shifts the focus of the class from the lecturer to me and is highly embarrassing—but I'm usually off again ten minutes later, and that tends to be my routine for the day.

Still, after nursing for almost eighteen years, I must have learned something. So I thought I would pass on a few pearls of wisdom on the subject of 'cooping' (verb: to sleep while at study).

Can I make it plain here and now that I am not advocating a mass nap for nurses on study days, but people do drop off—I'm just acknowledging the fact.

First, it must be stressed that we fall asleep for one of two reasons: fatigue or boredom. If you fall asleep because you're tired, then you can't help it. It's a law of nature. Everyone needs to sleep and it's not your fault that you need to sleep in the middle of an ENB 998 study day. Of course, if you drop off due to boredom then the lecturer is at fault, so no blame can attach itself to you there either.

So, you go into the classroom bright-eyed and bushy-tailed with no intention of sleeping, but by 9:30 AM you're ready for your milky drink and slippers. This is where Nick's Cooping Strategy comes in.

One: sit in the right place. This does not mean at the back where you will be picked on for those on-the-spot trick questions, which are difficult to answer when you are spending your lottery win on a Balinese beach while blowing sand off your coconut. Sit in the middle rows, off-centre to the lecturer. If he or she sits off-centre then sit on the same side. This reduces eye contact and pressure on you.

Two: do not sit next to Keen and Brainy or Thick and Slow as they might attract unwanted attention to you, so go for the intermediate set.

Three: if you have a desk, roll your sleeves up to make sure your elbows don't slide across the surface when you rest your chin in your hands.

Four: if possible, sit in chairs with a cloth upholstery rather than PVC. No matter how good you are at covering up your slumbers, you will be exposed when your body relaxes and you slide to the floor.

Five: if it is a lecture you are particularly interested in, give a trusted friend with legible handwriting some carbon paper.

Six: as lecturers become less imaginative, audio-visual aids are becoming increasingly common, which is good news for coopers. Dim lighting makes for an ideal cooping environment. A pillow would be nice, but instead try developing a soft, flabby forearm—it makes a perfectly adequate alternative.

If you have ever stayed awake during one of these videos then you will have noticed that the lecturer pays no attention to the screen and instead either stares out of the window, probing his ear with a pencil, or looks directly at you. If this happens, try leaning back in your chair to avoid his field of vision.

Despite all these tricks, occasionally you are going to come up against something unusual, something bizarre, something that keeps you awake despite your best efforts—the Interesting Lecturer. Thankfully, these days, they are few and far between, and anyway, who wants to go and spoil everything by making lectures interesting?

But is it Sterile?

Loretta Smith

In the midst of teaching sterile technique to two student nurses, a nursing instructor was called out of the room. I was behind the curtain, caring for another patient, when I heard the unmistakable sound of an instrument falling to the floor. The next thing I heard was the hushed voice of one of the students, telling the other, "Quick, pick it up before it gets contaminated."

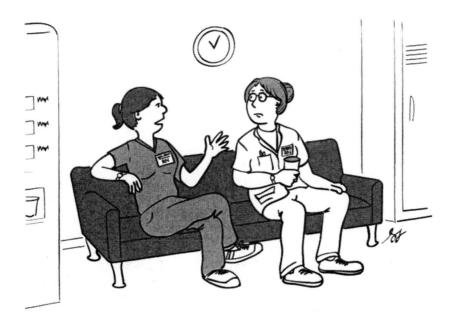

I can fullfill my CE credit from stories I hear around the hospital.

Stating the Obvious
Jane Tyke

What is it with research? It seems to me that as soon as anything new is published these days, everyone is gagging to change their practice in the name of evidence-based medicine. All on the whim of some lofty academics who wouldn't recognise an actual patient if they fell on them. Some studies are so mind-blowingly obvious you have to admire the gall of those who took the time, effort and perhaps taxpayers' money to point out what we already know.

I have a cutting in front of me from a recent medical journal and the headline proclaims "Avoiding fizzy drinks could prevent childhood obesity." Well, I wonder which brainbox thought up that one.

What about that study on hunted stags a few years ago? This brought about the amazing revelation that the poor beasts showed physical signs of high stress levels after being chased to the point of exhaustion and then caught. Nothing like stating the bleedin' obvious, in the words of Basil Fawlty.

Personally, I take a lot of research with a pinch of salt, especially the sort peddled by drug reps with a third class degree in media studies.

As professionals, we are expected to practice from a solid evidence base, but the goalposts keep shifting and what goes around, comes around. Take dietary advice. Back in my day, (the 1980s, not the 1880s as The Husband likes to wisecrack), diabetics in hospital were kept on strict, carbohydrate-controlled diets to control their sugars. It was a faff having to sort out all these special meals, but they worked. Anyone wanting to lose weight back then cut out bread and potatoes for a while and bingo, a more svelte silhouette. Then we were told to eat only low fat products and fill up on those healthy, energy-giving starches instead. Now, it's back to low carbs again, thanks to Dr Atkins and his billion dollar empire.

When I was a fairly senior midwife, new graduate criticised me for performing the fairly common practice of artificially rupturing membranes (ARM) in order to expedite labour. According to her, it was always wrong, no exceptions. Her mantra was: "But research shows..." which she tended to repeat ad nauseam. Yes, I conceded, ritual ARMs performed too early could complicate matters. However, according to my personal log of several hundred deliveries, a well-placed ARM worked a treat every time. In my experience, multiparous women in advanced labour often requested it in order to get the sprog out pronto.

Now, I have nothing against graduate nurses and midwives, I became one myself after a long, drawn out process. Like many nurses, I graduated after years of varied practice and increasing my knowledge base part-time, rather than with 3 years of theory. My point is, yes, we should take note of the new studies that are published, but with a critical eye. Never accept, always question. Your experience has to count for something, because you can't learn everything from books.

Perhaps I should do some proper research into this...?

Reprinted with permission from Practice Nurse, ©2004; 28(9): 17.

Keeping Them in Stitches: Humor in Perioperative Education
Janice M. Beitz, PhD, RN, CS, CNOR, CETN

One of the most fun activities I've started in recent years is the use of student and staff talent in generating humor for future educational use. One activity that has been productive is asking participants to devise funny book titles and brief stories that go with them. Some titles they've generated include:
- Tales From the OR Front Lines: The Good, the Bad, and the Bozos
- The OR Nurse's Manual: Or Everything I Knew About OR Nursing I Forgot by 9 AM

- Your Guide to Selecting a Good Surgeon: Or "A Cut Above"
- Your Guide to Selecting the Heavenly OR (Without Having to Visit)
- Humor—Don't Start the Case Without It
- The Illustrated History of Surgery (or The "Good Old Bad Old Days")
- Aging Ankles, Empty Mind: Confessions of an OR Nurse
- Fruitcakes Are Us: Your Professional Perioperative Team
- The Joy of Stress: An Advanced Perioperative Sourcebook

Reprinted from Seminars in Perioperative Nursing, ©1999; 8(2): 71-79 with permission from Elsevier. Edited from the original.

Bathing Beauty
Lisa Pitler, RN, OCN, MS

Soon after I learned how to give a bed bath, my instructor assigned me to bathe an elderly patient. When I entered the man's room, he seemed to be sleeping, so I quietly prepared what I needed and, with total concentration, set about gently washing him.

I was almost done when my instructor came in and asked if everything was going all right. I told her that my patient was quiet and seemed to be enjoying his bath.

She took me aside and pointed out that my patient had died several hours earlier. No wonder he'd seemed so peaceful.

Reprinted with permission from Journal of Nursing Jocularity.

Media Lament
Karen H. Morin, DSN, RN

I have seen too many well-known speakers present their visuals in a poor, distracting, or unprofessional manner. The following poem was written as a friendly, funny reminder to the reader to take care as they prepare and use visual aids.

Busy slides, oh no!
How could this be so?

Blank screen,
Unsightly scene,
Again and again.
Oh such pain!

Using transparencies
Without sensitivities
For one's eyesight
Oh, what a fright!

Illustrious speakers,
Established speakers,
Why such bleepers?

Is it that
They just don't know
How to show
Information to the best?
Or is the presenter in distress?

Ah, perhaps the problem is
Just not time
To do the job
Just fine!

Best Excuses if You Get Caught Sleeping at Your Desk

1. "They told me at the blood bank this might happen."
2. "This is just a 15 minute power-nap like they raved about in the last time management course you sent me to."
3. "Whew! Guess I left the top off the liquid paper."
4. "I wasn't sleeping! I was meditating on the mission statement and envisioning a new paradigm!"
5. "This is one of the seven habits of highly effective people!"
6. "I was testing the keyboard for drool resistance."
7. "Actually doing a "Stress Level Elimination Exercise Plan" (SLEEP) you learned at the last mandatory seminar your boss made you attend.
8. "I was doing a highly specific Yoga exercise to relieve work-related stress. Are you discriminatory towards people who practice Yoga?"
9. "Darn! Why did you interrupt me? I had almost figured out a solution to our biggest problem."
10. "The coffee machine is broke...."
11. "Someone must've put decaf in the wrong pot."

12. Boy, that cold medicine I took last night just won't wear off!"
13. "Ah, the unique and unpredictable circadian rhythms of the workaholic!"
14. "Wasn't sleeping. Was trying to pick up contact lens without hands."

Reprinted with permission. Retrieved June 27, 2005 from www.laughnet.net

Expert Nurse vs. Educated Nurse
Pat Veitenthal, RN, BSN

Expert Nurse	Educated Nurse
Has a résumé	Has a *Curriculum Vitae*
Can look at a child & pour correct dose of Tylenol	Has to weigh child, calculate mg/kg, then convert to ml
Can drop any size or type of tube past a pharynx	Can spell pharynx
Wipes up vomit and continues on	Waits for housekeeping to come
Sneaks phone advice so that people who don't need to be in the ER don't come in	Tells EVERYONE to come in
Uses lots of four letter words	Uses the word "inappropriate"
Can smell Cancer	Can cite Cancer statistics
Draws 6 tubes of blood off of one IV stick won't lose a drop	Calls lab & the IV team, or will have a HazMat spill
Wants the dose, route and frequency	Wants the *rationale*
Can "eyeball" the correct drip	Has to program a pump for a bolus factor rate
Watches *ER*	Watches *Chicago Hope*
Knows an MI when s/he sees one	Waits for CK and EKG results first
Ignores doctors, then *does* the right thing	Argues or corrects the doctors about *who's* right
Know when to ask for help	Should ask for help more often

Reprinted from Revolution: the Journal of Nurse Empowerment ©1996; 6(4): 77 with permission of the author.

Look for the Silver Lining 8

Restructuring, reengineering, and downsizing are not merely upheavals in the system that will eventually pass. These changes are fundamentally reshaping the relationship between management and employees forever. Nurses have to be flexible and ready to adapt to their roles within the organization to meet new demands and address emerging needs. What's more, an optimistic attitude and the ability to laugh at ourselves from time to time make it easier to relate personally and professionally. Never underestimate the value of having fun at work during your entire career.

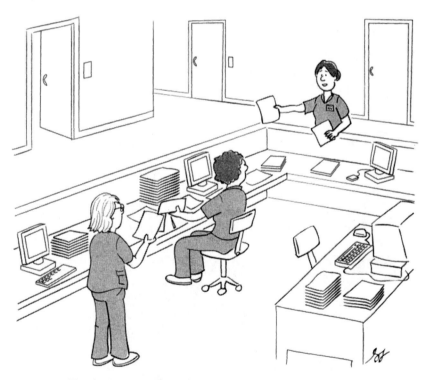

Here's one more form from management detailing all
the other forms we're supposed to fill out.

Modern Nurses Need a Perfect Body
Jo Brand

Over the past 10 years or so RNs have been taught through the use of those fascinating nursing models (fascinating in the sense of extremely dull, that is) not to treat patients like separate bits of bodies but to take a more holistic approach to care.

To solve the problem of nurse recruitment, however, I think it would be useful for us to break down nurses into their constituent parts to examine what the NHS is on the lookout for.

Let's start at the feet shall we? Nurses need to have feet that are in particularly good condition because, given current staffing levels, they are likely to be rushed off them. This is quite difficult to do while simultaneously keeping said feet firmly on the ground, but that is where they'll need to be.

Your skin also needs to be thick to deal with the backlash I sense is coming against nurses after the first rumblings of discontent in the media, which is discovering (knock me down with a soiled dressing, matron) that not all nurses are angels. And perhaps it is time for people to realise that nurses are ordinary people who are just as hurt by abuse as anyone else, rather than elasticated emotional punchbags who bounce back interminably.

This doesn't mean I'm advocating that the words 'shove off, you moron' should become a central part of the nursing vocabulary, but sometimes that forced smile feels like it's going to crack your face if you have to hold it through yet another insult.

Bosoms could perhaps be detachable for those days when female nurses come into contact with medical students. And anyone who thinks medical students are quite sweet should go to one of their balls and listen carefully to the heckling content. Incidentally, I suggest male nurses hang onto their balls—a definite requirement.

Eyes, of course, need to be propped wide open and preferably in the back of your head to do the job of two people at once. While we're in the head area, many people will say you need to have it examined if you want to go into nursing these days. But they'll be glad you're there when they need their heads examined in casualty on a Friday night after a close encounter of the 'Are you looking at my pint?' kind with the resident psychopath in their local.

Your brain, of course, needs to be able to perform many functions at once and yet immediately switch off from work when you are in the pub, so that the stresses of the day are not brought to bear upon an innocent old lady enjoying a Babycham.

Your elbows need to be nice and greasy—you'll need that grease on difficult days. And your back needs to be strong and broad as you may find you are constantly telling members of other disciplines to get off it as you try to get on with your work.

Make sure your nose is somewhere near that grindstone, your shoulder's to the wheel and all your hands are on deck. Once all these parts are working in harmony, you can cope with most things in the nursing profession.

Memorandum: Addendum to the Employee Handbook

To: All Employees
Subject: Sick Leave Policy

Sickness:

No excuse... We will no longer accept your doctor's statement as proof. We believe that if you are able to go to the doctor, you are able to come to work.

An operation:

We are no longer allowing this practice. We wish to discourage any thoughts that you may need an operation. We believe that as long as you are an employee here, you will need all of whatever you have and should not consider having anything removed. We hired you as you are, and to have anything removed would certainly make you less than we bargained for.

Death:

Other than your own: This is no excuse for missing work. There is nothing you can do for them, and we are sure that someone else can attend to the arrangements. However, if the funeral can be held in the late afternoon, we will be glad to allow you to work through your lunch hour and subsequently let you leave 1 hour early, provided your share of the work is ahead enough to keep the job going in your absence.

Your own: This will be accepted as an excuse. However, we require at least two weeks notice as we feel it is your duty to train your replacement.

Also:

Entirely too much time is being spent in the restroom. In the future, we will follow the practice of going in alphabetical order. For instance, those whose names begin with "A" will go from 8:00-8:15, and so on. If you're unable to go at your time, it will be necessary to wait until the next day when your time comes again.

We appreciate your cooperation,

THE MANAGEMENT
Reprinted with permission. Retrieved September 22, 2005 from www.carenurse.com

A Cost Saving Memo

Memorandum

To: All Hospital Employees
From: Administration
Effective immediately, this hospital will no longer provide security. Each Charge Nurse will be issued with a .38 caliber revolver and 12 rounds of ammunition. An additional 12 rounds will be stored in the pharmacy. In addition to routine nursing duties, Charge Nurses will patrol the hospital grounds 3 times each shift. In light of the similarity of monitoring equipment, the Critical Care Units will now assume security surveillance duties. The unit secretary will be responsible for watching cardiac and security monitors, as well as continuing previous secretarial duties.

Food service will be discontinued. Patients wishing to be fed will need to let their families know to bring them something, or make arrangements with Subway, Dominos, Wendy's, or another outside food preparation facility, prior to mealtime. Coin-operated telephones will be available in the patient rooms for this purpose, as well as for calls the patient may wish to make.

Housekeeping and Physical Therapy are being combined. Mops will be issued to those patients who are ambulatory, thus providing range of motion exercise, as well as a clean environment. Families and ambulatory patients may also register to clean the room of non-ambulatory patients for discounts on their bill. Time cards will be provided to those registered.

Nursing Administration is assuming the grounds keeping duties. If a Nursing Supervisor cannot be reached by phone or beeper, it is suggested to listen for the sound of the lawn mower, weed eater, or leaf blower.

Engineering will also be eliminated. The Hospital has subscribed to the Time-Life series of "How to..." maintenance books. These books may be checked out from Administration. Also, a toolbox of standard equipment will be issued to all Nursing Units. We will be receiving the volumes at a rate of one per month, and have received the volume on basic wiring. If a non-electrical problem occurs, please try to repair it as best as possible until that particular volume arrives.

Cutbacks in Phlebotomy staff will be accommodated by only performing blood-related laboratory studies on patients already bleeding.

Physicians will be informed that they may order no more than two (2) X-rays per patient per stay. This is due to the turn-around time required by the local Photomat. Two prints will be provided for the price of one and physicians are encouraged to clip coupons from the Sunday paper if more prints are desired. Photomat will also honor competitors coupons for one-hour processing in an emergency. If employees come across any coupons, they are encouraged to clip them and send them to the Emergency Room.

In light of the extremely hot summer temperatures, the local Electric Company has been asked to install individual meters in each patient room so that electrical consumption can be monitored and appropriately billed. Fans may be rented or purchased in the Gift Shop.

In addition to the current recycling programs, a bin for the collection of unused fruit and bread will soon be provided on each floor. Families, patients and the few remaining staff are encouraged to contribute discarded produce. The resulting moldy compost will be utilized by the pharmacy for nosocomial production of antibiotics. These antibiotics will be available for purchase through the hospital pharmacy, and will, coincidentally, soon be the only antibiotics listed in the hospital's formulary.

Although these cutbacks and changes may appear drastic on the surface, the Administration feels that over time we will all benefit from this latest cost cutting measures.

Reprinted with permission. Retrieved June 24, 2005 from www.nursinghumor.com

The Six Million Dollar Nurse
Jane Bliss-Holtz, DNSc, RN, BC

The good news is that job openings for nurses continue to grow (so we're likely to be employed for as long as we want), but the bad news is that those who choose the profession will continue to be faced with challenges of keeping their own health and well-being in perspective as they are called to work longer and increasingly more intense hours. Perhaps it is because I heard the other day that a movie based on the old "Six Million Dollar Man" television program is in the works, but I began to daydream about the possibilities of how technology like this could affect nursing. Just think—in the future... *faster... smarter... stronger... the cybernetically-genetically enhanced nurse.* I can see the news media reports now...

"C-GENS Continue to Be a Hit with Health Care"

No cold-hearted robot here; this cybernetically-genetically enhanced nurse (C-GEN for short) is fully human in all his/her attributes—just more so.

Faster

Replicating older time motion studies of the 2010 decade, studies into the 2030s have supported that continual refinement of older C-Gen enhancements make delivery of patient care treatments even faster and more cost effective. It has been found, however, that delivery of patient and family education still needs to be performed at a somewhat slower pace than other interventions, as health care consumers continue to need time to process health care information. It has been suggested that implantation of information microchips into patients may be the solution to this issue; however adding this procedure to the time spent in patient–nurse interface may not prove to be cost effective.

Smarter

Through biotechnology and continued genetic enhancement, time in academic preparation for a generic baccalaureate degree currently has been reduced to 12 months. Additionally, easily upgradeable neurochips have been standard equipment in C-GEN's since the early 2020s. This enhancement allows frequent changes in genetic and drug therapies and nursing treatment modalities to be added in a timely manner into the C-GEN's armamentarium of intervention strategies.

Critical-thinking (C-T) algorithmic neurogenic pathways have been in alpha and beta development for the C-GEN since 2015; however, there continue to be problems with development. One of the major issues is the inability to create sufficient algorithmic contingency bypasses to handle frequent overload from unanticipated variations in the health care environment. For example, beta-test of the most recent C-T pathway resulted in system shutdown when the prototype C-GEN was simultaneously presented with two new admissions, five stat physician orders, one hysterical postoperative toddler, two calls from radiology requesting a patient, and a sudden IV pump failure. Program developers continue to closely monitor non-C–GENs in an attempt to determine how they continue to avoid meltdown in similar scenarios.

Stronger

With titanium-sheathed vertebrae and flex-steel ligaments, C-GENs are able to transfer adolescents with full body casts and traction equipment from stretcher to bed with ease and minimum risk of self-injury. C-GENs are resistant to most of the common viruses that are found within health care settings and have been genetically programmed since 2020 to adapt to newer viral strains. One major flaw in the genetic program has been the continued failure to be able to protect the C-GEN from the virus that causes the "common cold." An unfortunate byproduct of C-GEN contact with this virus is that of cascade failure that eventually affects primary systems, resulting in a 7 to 10 day downtime. C-GEN technologists continue to study non-C–GENS to determine how they continue to function under the same conditions. It is predicted that there will be a breakthrough in this programming challenge by 2035....

Reengineering for the Birds
Darlene Sredl, RN, MA, MSN, PhD

Large institutions are routinely troubled by well-meaning, though weak-bladdered members of the Avian community. Sometimes, however, the institution itself is for the birds. Such is the case as we look in on Metropolis Health Center, just down the street from market-share rival, Our Lady of Perpetual Payment. We have a bird's eye view as they flock to the Hospital bored room, conveniently branched off the Administrative Roost.

It was obvious that the CEO did not want to go out on a limb by himself, or possibly lay an egg; so, he called the brood together to incubate the seed of a bold new Vulture—reengineering. The meeting began with some Flamingo dancers for light entertainment. "Call the Role. Where's your pen, Gwen?"

"Right here sir, ready to take down every word."

The pecking order included:

Robin Nightingale—Director of Nestlings
The Ruffled Grouse—Assistant Director of Nestlings
The Yellow-Bellied Sapsucker—VP (Operations)
The Humming Bird—Chief Financial Officer (CFO)
The Balding Corporate Legal Eagle
The Common Snipe Director of Security
The Southern Dodo Director of Maintenance
The Albino Peacock Director of Housekeeping
The Cockatoo—Assistant Director of Housekeeping
The Bare-Faced Buzzard—Director of Marketing
The Red-Necked Loon—Director of Psychiatry
And, of course, in the Captain's Nest, The Horn-Rimmed Owl, as CEO

The obfuscation began, "We are gathered together today to talk about reengineering and the new economic enterprise."

"You mean, Trekkies?" queried the CFO.

"The CFO must have seen a UFO!" quipped the Buzzard.

"Reengineering is the new buzzword, Buzzard.

We're talking about our new adversarial competitive strategy. First, we map out a framework for change and then we allocate appropriate resources to accomplish that change. Let's hear it from the Vice President. Which vice are you presiding over today?"

"Gift shop lottery sales are way off."

"Why?"

"I think somewhere in our employee manual it says you can't gamble while on duty."

"Hum-m-m..." mused the CFO. "To gambol means to walk around casually and with no definite purpose, doesn't it?"

"Yes sir!"

"Well, that describes most of our employees," ruffled the Grouse.

"Ok, so we will continue to prohibit loitering or casual walking. We will continue to prohibit gamboling on company time. The secretary just has to chickenscratch a few letters in the manual. No major rewrite. Now, back to the lottery sales—I want the gift shop profits up!"

"Why not let the employers use their ID badge like credit cards to make purchases?" suggested the Dodo.

"Oh, no, Dodo, are you suggesting we put it on their bills" Humm-m-m..." mused the Humming Bird.

"What multi-skilled pleuralistic thinking. What statistical congruence! That is the seed of a great idea!" screeched the owl. "Quack. Get it signed and witnessed by a Notary Republic."

"I think Democrats should have an equal say. After all, this is an election year"... mused the Wren.

"Figures for high performance employee resources must be bottomed out," the CFO continued.

"How are we going to do that?" challenged the Mocking Bird. "How are we going to find the personnel? The type of employee we seek is not going to work for chickenfeed."

"How do you screen potential new employees?" asked the CEO.

"Security runs a record chick. Many are afowl of the law. Some come straight from the pen" snipped the Snipe.

"Then," concluded the CFO, "Hire only jailbirds."

"What?"

"You said they're willing to work for scratch, didn't you? Besides, you could put peepers in their pockets so we would know where they are in case they're thinking of flying south and, we can buy their uniforms from Amber Crowbee and Finch."

"Well I can."

"What did you say?"

"The Pelican, we need a Pelican on our bored to oversea them."

"Remember, added the CEO, "fragmented operations focus functional barriers to the integrated processing systems that has downgraded this hospital's consumer applications."

"What does that mean, sir?" they cried in unison.

"My little chickadees, it means that the healthcare consumer is integral but unnecessary. Furthermore, the infrastructure we used to rely on can no longer empower or subjugate a breakdown in the chassis system so that the logarithm of success is as farfetched as ever. Are you all birdbrains?"

"Oh, thank you for explaining it sir," cheaped the CFO.

"Validation and construct integrity continue to dominate our vision, the CEO raled on.

"Do you need glasses, Sir?"

"Horn rims, remember?"

Let's consider the platform alternatives," continued the CEO.

"Running for President, Mr. President?"

"I'm talking about *artificial* intelligence."

"We've used that for years."

"I mean *Real* artificial intelligence."

"We prefer Apple Computers for the obvious reasons, of course."

"Outsource foodsource?"

"Yeah, Birdseye products."

"But, I deduced…"

"You could get arrested for that, sir" the Snipe interjected.

"But, the proposition must touch everyone…"

"There you go again, Mr. President." The Grouse's feathers ruffled.

"Don't you want to see the new digital system?" he asked the Ravenfeathered Nightengale.

"Not NOW, sir!"

"Spreadsheet?"

"Innuendo!"

"You would peck'er?"

"I object" thundered the legal eagle.

"On what grounds?"

"Habeus Corpus Luteum."

"Oh, Ok, OK. Back to the basics. Anticipate, initiate, precipitate. We cannot Parrot the past. That's a Cardinal sin. The key challenge? Abstractions and contradictions. Our minds must be open to any possibility including impossibility. I say, the values of this organization shall remain firm unless they become dispensable" the CEO warbled on.

"We can begin an excremental improvement program" offered the Director of Avian Resources.

"Hey, cleaning is my territory" squawked the Peacock.

"Preening, not cleaning is your territory" countered the Mocking Bird who continued, "For example, Sabbaticals. We could give employees three months off every seven years."

"But, current market research indicates the average avian lifespan just approaches 5.8 years."

"Exactly! We won't have to EsCrow any retirement.

What a savings," squawked the CFO.

"In conclusion, we must forge ahead with corporate competency and myopic instability. Overall, never remember to forget. We must end what we have begun and begin what must end. Teamwork will boldly rebuild the framework of the future and converge upon an axis of revolution. I say, Healthcare must.., not only molt, it must revolt..."

"Sir. It's already revolting!"

Reprinted from Journal of Irreproducible Results, www.jir.com, ©1998; 43(1): 16-17 with permission of the author. Edited from the original.

Arsenic and Old Remedies
Carrie Farella, RN, MA

First try coffee. Then try cannabis. If those don't work, reach for a trusty arsenic cigarette, and inhale it deeply. Thankfully, asthma treatments have come a long way in the last century.

Looking back at how patients were cared for 100 years ago conjures up images of cave people and dinosaurs. But at the time, prehistoric-like care was no laughing matter. Proving that medicine has a funny bone, Merck & Company, publishers of the famous *Merck Manual*, dusted off their first work, a slender volume, published 100 years ago, reprinting it just for fun.

Just 192 pages long, the work is chock-full of grins and giggles for anyone yearning to poke fun at mighty physicians and stuffy pharmacists of old. But be careful how hard you laugh—remember it was often a nurse who was administering the phoney baloney cures.

A spectrum of respiratory ailments plagued the people of 1899. Bronchitis could be treated with one of 80 different compounds and procedures. Most popular was belladonna (especially for children), a lethal compound that often killed patients who ingested it. Tar, used as a throat spray, was believed to lessen evil secretions. Devices were also popular. Bronchitis patients might be dressed in a stylish chamois waistcoat, belted oh-so-tightly to prevent mucous from pooling in the lungs. A lucky patient might be treated to an ice pack strategically placed on the lower spine. If that didn't stop the incessant coughing, bleeding patients from their jugular veins seemed to snap them back into shape—or kill them—whichever came first. Oddly enough, a patient's death certificate often read, "Died of bronchitis," and not "Died because he was put in a straight jacket, had his jugular veins sliced, and was strapped sitting to an ice bag." So much for documentation.

Obstetrics and gynecology also called for imaginative concoctions. Vague complaints related to pregnancy were treated with mercury, iodine, or chloroform water. The "nervous" gravid woman might be given caffeine, opium, or tasty lime salts. Once labor began, the woman could receive eucalyptus oil, belladonna, or the ever-popular powdered borax. No epidurals here, a sympathetic physician had cannabis and morphine handy. Thank goodness he had something in that little black bag.

The postpartum period was another area of womens' health that necessitated creative pharmacology. A new mother with "defective lactation ability" due to mastitis or breast abscesses received a castor oil rub or dry malt extract to sip. Nursing mothers diagnosed with "excessive lactation" nibbled parsley and endured a shock of electricity. Where was the La Leche League when we needed it?

Children who survived birth faced odd treatments. Babies with croup received "a splash of cold water dabbed in the face," a tartar emetic, or the lancing of their gums. Inhalers and nebulizers were the stuff of which dreams were made.

Patients with psychological impairments were treated especially well; "mania" including delirium, insanity, as well as the "puerperal mania," today's postpartum depression, received iron or digitalis. Many a psychiatric patient eagerly awaited a cold douche "to the head while the body is immersed in hot water." Elavil and Prozac were just a frustrated pharmacist's fantasy.

The year 1899 was also not the time to be a "convalescent." An elderly (50ish) person might have endured drinking cream, quinine tonics, and opium enemas—just the ticket for insomnia. Indeed, geriatric nursing has come a long way, baby.

In many cases, physicians were on the right track. Constipation, for example, was often relieved by eating whole-meal bread, prunes, licorice powder, or drinking water. If that failed, a "tobacco cigarette after breakfast," and a round of "gymnastics or horseback riding" often got things moving.

The end of a millennium is as good a time as any to reflect on the way things used to be. We can chuckle, sneer, and pretend we are so much more sophisticated than our counterparts of a century ago. But without the failed opium enemas, the tar throat spray deaths, and the arsenic overdoses, where would we be today? Even more frightening, in 2100, what will they say about us?

The Joys of Aging
Leslie Gibson, RN, BS

The Perks of Being Over 40
1. Kidnappers are not very interested in you.
2. In a hostage situation, you are likely to be released first.
3. No one expects you to run into a burning building.
4. People call at 9:00 PM and ask, "Did I wake you?"
5. People no longer view you as a hypochondriac.
6. There is nothing left to learn the hard way.
7. Things you buy now won't wear out.
8. You can eat dinner at 4:00 PM.
9. You can live without sex but not without glasses.
10. You enjoy hearing about other peoples' operations.
11. You get into heated arguments about pension plans.
12. You have a party and the neighbors don't even realize it.
13. You no longer think of speed limits as a challenge.
14. You quit trying to hold your stomach in, no matter who walks into the room.
15. You sing along with elevator music.
16. Your eyes won't get much worse.
17. Your health plan is beginning to pay off.
18. Your joints are more accurate meteorologists than the national weather service.
19. Your secrets are safe with your friends because they can't remember them either.
20. Your supply of brain cells is finally down to manageable size.
21. You can't remember who sent you this list.

Games for the Over-40 Crowd
1. Sag, You're It.
2. Pin the Toupee on the Bald Guy.
3. 20 Questions (shouted into your good ear).
4. Red Rover, Red Rover, the Nurse says Bend Over.
5. Doc Goose.
6. Simon Says Something Incoherent.
7. Hide and Go Pee.

8. Spin the Bottle of Mylanta.
9. Musical Recliners.

Signs of Menopause

1. You sell your home heating system at a yard sale.
2. Your husband jokes that instead of buying a wood stove, he is using you to heat the family room this winter. Rather than just saying you are not amused, you shoot him.
3. You have to write Post-It notes with your kids' names on them.
4. The phenobarbital dose that wiped out the Heaven's Gate Cult gives you 4 hours of decent rest.
5. You change your underwear after every sneeze.
6. You're on so much estrogen that you take your Brownie troop on a field trip to Chippendales.

Signs of Wear

"Old" Is When....

1. Your sweetie says, "Let's go upstairs and make love," and you answer, "Pick one; I can't do both!"
2. Your friends compliment you on your new alligator shoes, and you're barefoot.
3. A sexy babe catches your fancy, and your pacemaker opens the garage door.
4. Going bra-less pulls all the wrinkles out of your face.
5. You don't care where your spouse goes, just as long as you don't have to go along.
6. You are cautioned to slow down by the doctor instead of by the police.
7. "Getting a little action" means you don't need to take any fiber today.
8. "Getting lucky" means you find your car in the parking lot.

Reprinted from Urologic Nursing, ©2003; 23(6): 443-444 with permission of the author. Edited from the original.

Cuts by Any Other Name

Mark Radcliffe, RMN

Some time in 1983 fat people stopped being fat and became horizontally challenged. A few days later thin people, envious of this linguistic collision with physiology, demanded the right to become horizontally reluctant. Bald people removed their hats to become follically subdued. Short people, sorry, vertically restrained people, were forced to stop taunting old lanky legs from down the road and instead recognise that he was, in fact, vertically unlimited.

Of course not everything changed: people who wear Crimplene remain fashionably unacceptable and health service managers are still really annoying.

The intention of modern language is to render words meaning— and value-free. Indicative of this is the fact that we have no desire to address social inequality; instead, we seek to make inequality more conversationally palatable. The health service is not immune. Purchasers, policy-makers and managers have embedded themselves in the language of alleged neutrality and invented a sackful of phrases to disguise content and sweeten the bitterest pill.

The pill is not sweetened and the content is plain to see. We know, for example, that 'decommissioning a service provision' is 'closing' but has more syllables. We also know that 'a period of consultation to review the commissioning intention of this authority' means 'closing but I have yet to write the memo.'

'A structural review of clinical grading requirements' means 'let's get rid of the G-grades.' If you hear that there is going to be an 'audit of the task breakdown and efficiency of day-to-day work patterns' then in reality there is a plan to persuade under-age immigrants to make beds and take blood pressure. And, of course, 'the need to relocate services to a more appropriate and accessible area' means 'we are moving your ward to a really cheap warehouse beside the bus garage.'

Language equivocates. That is part of its beauty. However, it does us no harm to examine the subtext that so affects our professional paradigm. The most offensive elements of health manager speak is its tendency to allude to a shared responsibility and assured progress. Let's face it, there is nothing progressive about talking like a failed Californian salesman with a thesaurus up his bottom.

What is wrong with these people? Do they really think that when they speak of 'service integration' we do not know they mean they are going to shut down the ward next door and move all the patients in here?

Amid all this nonsense there remain some phrases that, to the best of my knowledge, do not actually mean anything—for example, 'person-centred perspectives,' 'mapping outcome outlines' and 'multi-need response provision.'

Someone uses a ridiculous phrase like that and you cannot help but stop and wonder what the hell he or she is going on about. In that split second, the manager-type person sees that your guard is down and slips in something about 'decommissioning,' 'redundancy initiatives' or 'customer rationalisation' (death). It also gives the person time to leave the room before you deploy a coronation-style activity with a waste-disposal unit.

One of the most irritating and recurring phrases used is CRES. This is an abbreviation for 'cash-releasing efficiency saving' which, in turn, is an abbreviation for cuts. Other abbreviations for cuts include 'investment rationalisation,' 'a downturn in service development,' 'downsizing personnel capacity' and the perennial favourite 'correlating market appropriate spending initiatives in the public sector downloading pool.'

The most stressful circumstance that thousands of nurses find themselves in every day is one in which they have responsibility but very little power. Nurses frequently find themselves responsible for patient well-being, safety and maintenance.

But purchasers and managers are able, by employing the language of neutrality, to avoid the implications of their policies. They are faceless and blameless and their language protects them. 'Service integration' sounds so much nicer than 'closure,' 'rationalisation of care commitments' much cleaner than 'we will not provide the resources to meet all the needs, so it's up to you to choose who receives your attention.'

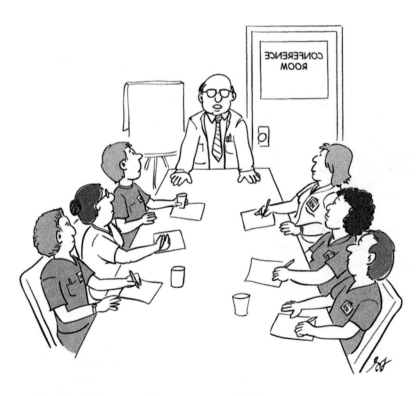

I have good news and bad news. The bad news is there is no cure for Mrs. Bates. But the good news is that the latest research indicates that laughter is still the best medicine.

How to Know You Are Growing Older
Leslie Gibson, RN, BS

- Everything hurts and what doesn't hurt, doesn't work.
- The gleam in your eye is from the sun hitting your bifocals.
- You feel like the night before and you haven't been anywhere.
- Your little black book contains only names ending in MD.
- Your children begin to look middle aged.
- A dripping faucet causes an uncontrollable bladder urge.
- You need glasses to find your glasses.
- You turn out the lights for economic rather than the romantic reasons.
- Your knees buckle but your belt won't.
- Your back goes out more than you do.
- You have too much room in the house and not enough in the medicine chest.
- You sink your teeth in a steak, and they stay there.
- YOU WONDER WHY MORE PEOPLE AREN'T USING THIS SIZE PRINT.

Reprinted from Urologic Nursing, ©2004; 24(4): 355-356 with permission of the author. Edited from the original.

Identity Crisis
Jane Tyke

Yet another enthusiastic PCT directive has bounded in, like a playful puppy on the rampage. Do they really think that we, at the cutting edge of saving lives, have time to read this drivel, let alone adhere to it? I suppose sending out these pearls of wisdom is giving someone meaningful employment and keeping them from the dole queue, but really, have they nothing else to do up at Ivory Towers?

This particular missive demands that all staff are to wear ID badges, as they do in the acute trust. Admittedly, in hospitals there is a bewildering array of personnel for patients to grapple with, but not so here. Just receptionists, nurses and GPs, whom most of the patients have known for donkeys' years anyway. No doubt if we all came in wearing badges there would be some witty comments about our inability to remember our own names.

In the workplace, staff are usually distinguishable by uniforms, official or otherwise. In hospitals you can tell the junior doctors by their ever-so-white coats bulging with stethoscopes, bleeps and dog-eared BNFs. Lofty consultants favour suits and dicky bows.

Senior nurses with daft titles like 'Acting clinical nurse manager' and 'Deputy quality assurance facilitator' wear sandwich boards, as there aren't badges large enough to do them justice. Lucky old OTs and physios get to parade round in fetching polyester trouser suits. Go to any psychiatric unit and you can identify the staff because they are more 'right-on' than their 'clients', sporting their myriad body piercings and carefully assembled scruffiness.

Back home in general practice, doctors are recognisable by their garish, breakfast-stained ties or Indian print frocks with sensible shoes. Many practice nurses wear the standard navy blue garb to prevent their own clothes being pebble dashed by various body fluids. I can't see the GPs kow-towing to this memo, and nor shall I. Dr Sarky, of course, expects everybody to know who he is and Dr Eager's shiny halo gives her away. But let's use some common sense here. Patients coming to see me get one or two clues on the way. First, they book the appointment with me. Then they are heartily summoned by reception, "Mrs Windbag to Sister Tyke, please! Last dungeon on the left!"

On arrival at the rabbit hutch masquerading as a consulting room, there is my name on the door, in large letters. Ah, but what about those who can't read it, I hear you ask. Well, panic not, for when they enter the room I introduce myself and make sure that they are the patient I am expecting.

So what good would a minuscule piece of plastic pinned on my chest do them? They would spend their precious ten-minute slot squinting at the tiny text instead of getting to the point.

I don't want all and sundry gawping at my left breast, thank you. I can get that kind of attention any night down at The Fursty Ferret!

Reprinted with permission from Practice Nurse, ©2004; 28(3): 47.

Rear View
Mark Radcliffe, RMN

You may have heard that there is a new breed of nurse (yes, another one) coming, and the powers that be have drafted in no less a national resource than psychologists to help select them.

Apparently, as part of the government's relentless drive towards getting nurses to be a bit more like doctors—but cheaper—new nurses called 'first-contact practitioners' are to be recruited and trained to perform 'medical duties' in general practice.

However, in order to decide what candidates are able to make the difficult decisions a medico-nurse will have to make, psychologists have invented a test that will tell us about the courage, initiative and resilience of the candidate. No one has yet suggested that candidates for medical school should undergo this test but then they usually have good A-level chemistry, so probably don't need that other stuff.

Two interesting things are happening here, the most important being the ongoing reinvention of nursing. The other one is confirmation that psychologists are trying to take over the world.

Everywhere we look these days there is a psychologist offering us tiny truths about everything from modern celebrity to international terrorism.

I recently watched a programme about some bloke who was afraid of heights and wanted to conquer his fear by doing a parachute jump. Cue Doctor Useless. "Your fear is your only enemy," the psychologist lied, clearly neglecting to mention gravity. And the poor sod jumped, which is not surprising really, given that he was being followed by a film crew and his 60-year-old mother who had offered to jump with him.

The psychologist closed the show with this searing insight into the nature of fear: "Sometimes you can overcome it, sometimes you can't. Where's my cheque?"

We have an ongoing quest in our house to find any documentary on anything from *Pop Idol* to problems in the Middle East that doesn't have a sassy psychologist at some point telling us that: "Human beings need to be loved/fed/danced with/occupied. Where's my cheque?"

Psychology is the new religion. All you have to do is believe and life will take care of itself; have faith in their insights and they will find the best nurses for us. I swear sometimes this country is becoming one great big cult.

Let's consider these new nurses—the ones with the right psychological profile, the quasi-medical training and the postgraduate qualification in crisis management. What is it about them that makes them a nurse? It seems the only thing that makes this a nursing role is the fact that it is someone who sees a patient but isn't quite a doctor.

Of course there is a strong argument that says such things don't really matter. After all, the health service requires a workforce that is able to respond to different needs in new and inventive ways. If nursing can demonstrate itself to be flexible then that is to its credit, isn't it?

Well maybe, except who says that nursing chooses the direction that it goes in? And who says that the core role of nursing—which I would describe as 'the social and material manifestation of human compassion'—is any less vital now than it ever has been?

I am not suggesting that there isn't a role for whatever a 'first-contact practitioner' is. There are probably all sorts of roles to illustrate the modernisation of the health service. But I don't quite understand what stops them from being new and specific roles.

Let them hang out with the allied health professionals playing Ker-Plunk and taking the mickey out of the psychologists. Loathe as I am to make a crass metaphor, if the health service is a car then nurses are the wheels, and if you keep reinventing the wheel it will eventually stop going round.

30 Thoughts for 30 Years
Sherry Anne Holden, RN, BSN

1. The work of your hands is more than a job, practice, or profession; your calling is a gift that should be handled with care.
2. Self-evaluation produces the best results.
3. Learn something new every day.
4. It's okay to say, "I don't know."
5. Be kind to one another. Great minds and exceptional talent are wasted for lack of kindness.
6. Touch is an art. Holding a hand, wiping a tear, and giving a hug transcend all else in a world of hurt.
7. You own your practice. Be accountable and responsible.
8. Reading the *Florence Nightingale Pledge* regularly will give you roots.
9. Create laughter and cultivate joy. It's good for everyone.
10. Strive to achieve a nurse/physician relationship based on professional respect and trust.
11. Mop a brow; mop a floor. Be flexible enough to meet the demands of any situation.
12. Hold fast to what's good. Sometimes we change so quickly that we lose sight of who and what we are.
13. The big rewards in nursing are never monetary in nature.
14. Power: Don't abuse it if you've got it.
15. Knowledge is power, but it's worthless unless shared.
16. Sometimes New Year's Day falls on January 5 and Thanksgiving in October. Your job will dictate holidays; your family will adjust.
17. Hospital management is a thankless job.
18. We lost a part of our identity when white uniforms and caps disappeared.
19. Pay attention to details.
20. The hospital environment is a chain of interdependency. A physician couldn't function efficiently without a nurse, and

a hospital would be useless without a cook or janitor. Sometimes we think more highly of ourselves than we ought.

21. Those who work the night shift are saintly.
22. Computers are here to stay. You don't have to like them, but you have to use them.
23. Regardless of computer technology, paperwork is never-ending.
24. Technology and ethics are strange bedfellows indeed.
25. Patients entrust their lives to us. Never take that responsibility lightly.
26. If you make a choice that's not right for you, make a change.
27. Forget the buzzwords you hear—empowerment, interfacing, convergence, restructuring. Focus on care.
28. Find something good in everyone
29. Prayer can influence healing.
30. The healing of a body is a continuous wonder. Remember, you're a small, but crucial, part of that miracle.

Reprinted with permission from Nursing 98, ©1998; 28(1): 32hn8.

I'm Too Old for This!
Pat Veitenthal, RN, BSN

There comes a time in a nurse's career when she says out loud what she's been saying to herself for years: I'm too old for this!

After 28 years, mostly in the emergency department, I'm old and tired and I hurt, mentally and physically. Don't get me wrong. I can still keep up, and I can even still dazzle on occasion, but the point is, I'm not sure I *want* to anymore.

Some of us have more trouble than others admitting this. In the early '70s, for example, I worked with a nurse who had only five digits in her Social Security number, yet she simply refused to retire. I can assure you, it was not a pretty sight watching her go from Super Nurse to Stupor Nurse. I don't want that to happen to either you or me, so here are some warning signs that will give you, roughly, a five-year warning.

You Know It's Almost Time to Retire If:
1. You refer to your colleagues as "The kids I work with."
2. Your work shoes are older than the doctor on duty.
3. You have to cross your legs before you can laugh at something funny.
4. You have to stop and think (which is okay), or you forget to start again (that's not okay).

5. You are exhausted after a code when you were the documentation nurse.
6. One day you say, 'Really? Me too!" to every patient you take care of.
7. You are not afraid to call the CEO by his first name—or at home.
8. You hold the door open for patients who want to go AMA (against medical advice) rather than argue.
9. They find old equipment in the basement, and call you to tell them what it is.
10. You think Managed Care is the name of a nursing home chain.

Reprinted from Revolution: the Journal of Nurse Empowerment, ©1996; 6(2): 89 with permission of the author.

Author Index

CPSIA information can be obtained
at www.ICGtesting.com
Printed in the USA
FFOW04n0301201217
44165530-43557FF